THE OHASHI BODYWORK BOOK

Beyond Shiatsu with the Ohashiatsu® Method

OHASHI

Photographs by Kan Okano

KODANSHA INTERNATIONAL

New York ◆ Tokyo ◆ London

OTHER BOOKS BY OHASHI:

Do-It-Yourself Shiatsu
Natural Childbirth the Eastern Way
Reading the Body: Ohashi's Book of Oriental Diagnosis
Touch for Love: Shiatsu for Your Baby
Zen Shiatsu (with Masunaga)
The Big Book of Relaxation (contributor)

VIDEOS BY OHASHI:

Art of Ohashi, Part 1: Back-Front Position
Art of Ohashi, Part 2: Side Position
Art of Ohashi, Part 3: Sit-Up Position
Art of Ohashi, Part 4: Neck Technique
Ohashiatsu® for a Healthy and Happy Pregnancy

Kodansha America, Inc.
114 Fifth Avenue, New York, New York 10011, U.S.A.

Kodansha International Ltd.
17-14 Otowa 1-chome, Bunkyo-ku, Tokyo 112, Japan

Published in 1996 by Kodansha America, Inc.

Library of Congress Cataloging-in-Publication Data
Ohashi, Wataru. The Ohashi bodywork book: beyond Shiatsu with
the Ohashiatsu method/Ohashi; photographs by Kan Okano.
p. cm.
ISBN 1-56836-096-7 (pbk.)
1. Acupressure—Handbooks, manuals, etc. 2. Acupressure points—Handbooks, manuals, etc. I. Title
RM723.A27033 1996
615.8'22—dc20   96-25898

Book design by Matthew Van Fleet

Printed in the United States of America

96 97 98 99 00 Q/KP 10 9 8 7 6 5 4 3 2 1

CONTENTS

INTRODUCTION

The Bible chronicles how Jesus Christ placed his hands on sufferers to heal them. Healing with the hands has been found around the globe for centuries, in cultures from those of Native Americans and Africans to those of colonial Rome. The *laying on of hands* is a universal concept, a natural human instinct. When you have a headache, you put your hands on your head and rub; if you have lower back pain, you put your hands on your back and press. This was the beginning of shiatsu (therapy given by applying pressure to points on the body), acupuncture, and other healing methods of Eastern cultures. You press, and then you find that pressing one point is more effective than pressing another. Soon you notice that some points actually form lines—those are meridians. Then you notice that the pressure is not strong enough, deep enough, so you use sharper instruments, such as bamboo sticks. Eventually, you realize that pressing with sticks is not deep enough, so you make devices to puncture the skin—acupuncture.

Oriental healing developed naturally, not in a scientific laboratory. Many practitioners, however, like to give the impression that shiatsu is a theoretical science, as a way of establishing their own so-called scientific wisdom. But any bodywork is intuitive, experiential, relying on natural instinct and behavior first. If people pay too much attention to theory, they soon start following the theory instead of the body; they give shiatsu from the brain only, and both givers and receivers suffer.

The concept of bodywork applies to all the techniques and methods used to manipulate or massage someone's body: physical therapy, chiropractic, massage, shiatsu, reflexology, and many others. Most practitioners use many techniques and sometimes more than one method. For them, bodywork is first of all *work*—they are working hard on someone else's body. All the effort is for the benefit of the receiver. Virtually every one of the hundreds of books I have read emphasizes how to deal with the receiver's problems, how to care for and cure, but say hardly a thing about the giver's well-being, the giver's consciousness, the giver's reward.

This book has been written for givers. The primary difference between the Ohashiatsu method and other bodywork methods is that Ohashiatsu maintains and improves the giver's posture, movement, and well-being. Priority must go to the practitioner. When you give Ohashiatsu, you get regenerated and energized because of the way your body moves, because you are enhancing your vital (ki) energy, and because you are meditating while you are working. Whose health would not improve with this type of exercise daily!

During the last thirty years, I have seen many a giver damage his or her body. While rescuing other people's bodies, practitioners ruin their own through bad posture, bad technique, bad movement, and unnatural force. When I observe other bodywork methods or read other books, especially on shiatsu, I first ask myself whether you, the practitioner, can really give five to ten treatments a day using these techniques, and can practice such treatment regularly for twenty years or more. Sooner or later, you must get tired; sooner or later, you will destroy your own body. You cannot give healthy bodywork unless you *have* a healthy body. If you don't mind your own body, how can you mind others' bodies?

I am small in stature, and I was born weak and unhealthy in my native Japan. This is fortunate. If I had been strong and had a big body and muscle power, I might not have developed my method. When I came to America after studying traditional shiatsu in Japan, I was at a disadvantage because of the size differential between Americans and me, so I had to think about how to utilize my disadvantage, how to turn my disadvantage to my advantage. If I had continued to practice shiatsu in my native country on small-bodied Japanese people, I wouldn't have needed to adapt. But here in America, I would have been destroyed by the size differential within a couple of years, so I had to change everything I had learned in the traditional method. Traditional shiatsu is not for givers. You learn how to press, where to press, how much to press. But given my size and strength limitations, this was not possible here. So the first principle of Ohashiatsu—don't press—came out of the relationship between Americans and me.

Besides being small and weak, I am also lazy. I am always asking myself how *not* to do things and what *not* to do; this is one reason I can be so effective. If you carefully avoid doing most things, in the end there are only one or two things you can do in a day—and you do those one or two things very effectively. But if you are strong and resolute and have lots of energy, you become obsessed with how much you can do and end up feeling inferior because you can't do what you had hoped. Working too hard wastes energy; being lazy focuses it.

This concept is hard for most Westerners to embrace. Many people who work hard don't achieve very much. They are scattered—not only in bodywork, but also in their own lives. If they sat down to meditate for half an hour or an hour, doing nothing would purify their effectiveness; it would not be wasting time, and in the end they would reap the benefit. This is why I am so confident that anybody who reads this book can do far better than I can. If someone with my disadvantages of being small, weak, and lazy can do so well, anyone else can do at least as well.

In Ohashiatsu, my body is in a state of complete tonus, which means relaxed and in a state of readiness for any demand. I don't tense anything; I don't press. In Ohashiatsu—as in t'ai chi, as in meditation—I am just *being*. Other bodywork techniques are *doing* techniques; Ohashiatsu is a *being* technique. I don't need to *do* anything. I just bring my body in line with the receiver's body, and then even my small body is more than enough. I learned this from meditation and from the Japanese self-defense art of aikido. The concept of aikido is nonresistance: Don't fight back. In boxing or wrestling, you need big muscles to meet a big body. But in aikido, you use your opponent's body, use his momentum, against him. This concept is also used in Ohashiatsu.

All bodyworkers, both amateurs and professionals, can benefit from this technique. First, you are getting older and eventually you won't have the body you have now; second, how many effective treatments could you give in one day using just your muscles? You would quickly tire. One of the principles in Ohashiatsu is *Be natural*. Being natural means that you must be very comfortable doing every single thing you do. Don't do anything that does not feel naturally comfortable. Don't pretend you're a master. Don't show off. Ohashiatsu is about being, not doing.

I came to the United States to attend graduate school in American literature, not to be a professional healing practitioner. In my mind I am still an amateur—not a master, not a professional. Professional therapists can become handicapped by the attitude that nobody else can do what they do; that only people with a special talent, and only after long study, can perform their kind of body-

work. This attitude then takes them further away from whatever brought them to bodywork in the first place. Because I started with an amateur's point of view, I was never attached to any one school of thought, and it is still possible for me to give up whatever does not work. I define and change and evolve all the time. I make joy, not obligation, my first priority.

Aikido, t'ai chi, meditation, Eastern healing philosophy, ballet, dance, mime, music, Zen: Ohashiatsu is the fruit of the versatility of my study and experience. Evolved from a base of traditional Japanese shiatsu, it differs from traditional shiatsu in the attitude of the giver, in the way techniques are utilized, and in the importance of using two hands. Like shiatsu and other Eastern therapies, it is a method that manipulates the energy within the body and uses a framework of Eastern philosophy. However, the emphasis of Ohashiatsu is on communication and synergism between giver and receiver; on the self-development of the giver as well as the receiver; and on true physical, psychological, and spiritual harmony for both. Further, my approach improves and preserves the giver's body, so that he or she can continue this wonderful work for many fruitful years.

Some bodywork methods are bland and empty because there is no personality in them. I believe that good bodywork must have a specific flavor and great dignity. I don't care for generic names, which no one takes responsibility for, so that is why my name is attached to Ohashiatsu. I don't want to call it *energy work*; I don't want to call it *shiatsu*; I don't want to call it *massage*. I've given it my own personality and character, and I take all the responsibility.

In the United States, the more famous and popular shiatsu becomes, the more it is being destroyed. Some people study shiatsu in a two-weekend course, then start charging for so-called "shiatsu" massage. Too often, traditional shiatsu is taught in a mechanical way with no attention to bodywork as art. Art is personal, not objective, nor can it be learned in a short time. It is only because Ohashiatsu is a personal art that it works. The basic framework of my practice is always evolving, always enlarging. Because I have had a variety of teachers, I am not limited to one approach.

Only recently did I begin teaching my philosophy and techniques in Japan—and while there, I taught in English that was then translated by others into Japanese. Were I to teach in Japanese, the students would have neither respected my approach to what they know as shiatsu, nor would they have appreciated its differences from the traditional method. Having lived in America for 25 years, I am Japanese, but I am also *not* Japanese from their point of view. When traditional knowledge returns to its source in a changed form, it must be presented in a different way. The very idea of self-development is an American one, not at all Japanese. The term *shiatsu* happens to be Japanese, but the practice of healing through touch is not exclusively Japanese. Ohashiatsu is universal. Because I have been teaching in the United States since 1972, and in England and Europe since 1976, training numerous students who eventually became teachers, Ohashiatsu is now being taught in Europe, North and South America, and Japan.

Many people believe that they have to achieve results under any circumstances, but your first priority should be to enjoy what you are doing. If you force yourself to do bodywork in spite of pain, your body will betray you or rebel against you.

You must also be endlessly curious about every aspect of your life while you practice. I am interested in philosophy, history, music, art, and dance—not just medical or technical information.

In fact, in the end, technique is just a small part of treatment. After a while, people no longer come for the technique, but for you, your personality, and your qualities as a human being, not only as a therapist.

Unfortunately, the longer I practice and the more well-known I become, the more people see me as a professional or a therapist or a master, and I have to work all the harder to deny it; if I accept their view of me, I will lose my joy, my potential to become better, and my original reason for starting to study. Many schools, many teachers, forget the importance of joy in learning, and they become preoccupied with knowledge and expertise only.

You may wonder how you can avoid "becoming a professional" and still do something in a serious way. This is a dilemma. To develop the best technique, to achieve your highest standard, you must be professional; but you also have to avoid the ego of professionalism. The key is in your attitude, your willingness to question professionalist pride while maintaining high standards. As long as you have a questioning spirit and an openness to self-development, you can avoid the professionalist pitfalls.

Every single day you are developing, improving. Your receiver is your teacher. Your receiver is your examiner. Your receiver is your assessor. Every session, every person, every day, is your own board of examiners. With this kind of attitude, you're always excited, you never get bored.

Don't Put Off Until Tomorrow

I have heard some people say, "I have to wait until I become healthy to give treatments to other people." I say that you will never become healthy if you wait. Waiting is a good excuse not to take care of yourself, so start while you are sick. Perhaps in maneuvering your body you will discover that you are not as bad off as you thought. Try Ohashiatsu especially when you are feeling fragile, when you have a headache or arthritis or lower back pain—or even cancer. Ohashiatsu is for the giver who wants to be healthy.

I have a student who is HIV positive. He told me that he had an arrogant and casual attitude toward life before becoming infected; afterward, he started to study and practice Ohashiatsu and discovered how deeply he appreciates every moment of life. Even though he has HIV, he is still alive and he has energy—he has *intention*. Of course, he is very ill but he still has the ability to enjoy life, to help others. *Ohashiatsu is for givers* means that when you are tired or sick, you should study and practice. When I am tired, I give sessions. Afterward, I feel wonderful.

If you follow the teachings of this book carefully, you will never get tired. Ohashiatsu is an energizing dance. It will aid in your recovery as much as meditation, exercise, or sleeping will. If you feel tired after you give Ohashiatsu, then you are not doing it correctly. If you don't feel happy after you give ten treatments a day, you are doing something wrong.

Of course, the receiver, too, benefits. Ki energy (the force that gives us life) is an essential part of health. And it is a mutual issue: When the giver enjoys, the receiver benefits, because he or she will open up his or her body more. Then, because the receiver naturally opens up more and is more comfortable, diagnosis is easier—making treatment easier and the result greater. Equally important, when as a giver you communicate your enjoyment and attitude about life to the receiver, the receiver will use your example to make him- or herself healthier and happier in the future. In Ohashiatsu, the giver is a model to the one receiving treatment, an example of how to live one's life and take care of one's health. It is as much a matter of personal development as it is of body training.

It has taken me more than 20 years to write this book, because I am still studying, still changing. Each day I discover something to improve my technique; you cannot refine technique overnight. Twenty years from now, I may want to write another book, but that possibility does not make me hesitant to publish this book now, because after decades of practicing, I am convinced that even now I am doing something right.

I want you to appreciate this book not only now, but also after years of practicing—correctly, naturally, effectively, and effortlessly. If you want to be a happy practitioner for years and years, you must develop good habits now. Sincere and dedicated bodyworkers become successful, and they become busier and busier, but after a few years of combining faulty techniques with too much devotion to work, they can do irreparable harm to themselves. They are still committed, but they cannot continue.

In Ohashiatsu, before you start giving bodywork, you should have an appreciation and awareness of your own health and well-being. Your focus should be on taking care of *your* health.

Many people misunderstand this approach; they say they want to sacrifice their lives to rescue other people who are suffering. Bodyworkers who hold to this belief frequently find that their techniques don't yield encouraging results, because the givers are working so hard to *do* that they get exhausted. Most bodyworkers discontinue their careers sooner or later precisely because they did sacrifice themselves to help other people.

Too many people do not see that sacrificing oneself is a type of arrogance. If I feel I am sacrificing myself to heal someone, I may want that person to admire me or be grateful to me. I may want to be recognized as a healer or to be called a psychic with special energies and talents. When I feel I am working so hard, sacrificing so much, my ego starts telling me, "You should be famous, successful, wealthy; your clients must compliment you and be grateful." In the end, you will come to depend on the compliment, and you will work even harder, sacrifice even more. It is important to guard against this type of thinking, and I warn my students often of its dangers: If you think you are working too hard helping other people, then you will also think you are suffering too much. Eventually, this kind of thinking will destroy the pure attitude you started with.

Ohashiatsu is for givers means it is not my business whether the receiver is getting healthy or not. Some receivers may get better, but I definitely get better. You, the giver, must not believe you are curing people, that you have psychic power, special energies, or healing abilities. You have no need for such claims when you already enjoy what you are doing. If your primary focus is on making the receiver better, you are expending energy in the wrong way; and if the receiver does not get better (some people resist being well), you will truly suffer.

Please study this book carefully and practice the techniques in it. If you enjoy what you are doing, you will want to do more, an attitude that is more spiritual than sacrificial, and in the end, you will help more people.

Other books may give you more detailed information, more philosophy and theory, or more techniques, but this book will help you be a happy giver for as many years as you choose to practice.

HOW TO USE
THIS BOOK

This book is intended primarily for givers—for those who want to learn to practice Ohashiatsu, as well as for those already practicing, who want to improve their technique. Most bodywork books focus on the receiver—on his or her condition and symptoms and the procedures for treating them; this may be the first book written for the giver. As a result, there is less detailed information here than in some of the other literature about meridian lines and tsubo points, how they relate to various parts of the body, and which to press for various complaints, because I believe that if givers pay attention to their own bodies, if they are well-balanced and comfortable, they will naturally be more sensitive to receivers.

I do, however, provide you with basic information for diagnosis and treatment. Included with this volume is a separate insert about the 14 meridians. It contains charts that map the locations of the meridians and the major tsubos (pressure points) along them, with a brief description of their functions, and it also contains a diagram of the areas where the meridians intersect the hara, the area between the rib cage and pelvic bones. The insert is designed so that you can keep it visible while you are practicing the techniques in this book, most of which follow the paths of the meridians. Don't be too concerned in the beginning about whether you are at exactly the right point on a meridian at any given time; it is enough at first to have a general idea of location and direction, and to focus instead on your own movement. You will develop your skills of diagnosis and treatment better by cultivating a responsive touch and attitude than by referring anxiously to a chart. If you stay in tonus and move naturally and continuously, you will be able to sense how much pressure to give for the greatest benefit of the receiver.

Once you feel you have mastered your own movement and the basic principles of diagnosis and treatment, you may want to learn more about how to evaluate the receiver's condition and how the meridians relate to different aspects of our health, for which I refer you to my earlier book, *Reading the Body*, which is devoted entirely to the subject of diagnosis. For further information about meridians and tsubos, I recommend my first book, *Do-It-Yourself Shiatsu*.

Part I of the present book outlines the basic principles and preparation for Ohashiatsu. Since this book emphasizes the bodywork of the giver, you should begin your study with the kata section (Chapter 2), which has exercises to help you learn balance, support, flexibility, and continuity. Repeat these exercises until the positions and movements have become almost instinctive, and then you will be ready to work on a receiver. (The kata exercises are good for your own well-being, whether you go on to practice Ohashiatsu or not.)

Part II presents techniques I have developed during 25 years of practice. You will never use all of them in any one treatment session—that would take at least four hours, which is far too long for a session. Even if you tried to use half of them, two hours of treatment is still too long. For a basic one-hour Ohashiatsu session, you need only a quarter of the techniques in this book. But practice them all, try to master them all, at your own

rate and according to your own condition. None are strictly for beginning or advanced students: Start with the techniques that are easiest for you and gradually go on to the ones that are more difficult. I cannot tell you which is which; degree of difficulty varies from person to person.

You will also note that I have included many examples of *wrong* techniques in *Don't* boxes. They illustrate the most common errors in body position and movement I have encountered during my years of teaching. The boxed material in the pages that follow offers tips, reminders, and warnings or demonstrates ways to use your body that may be applicable to more than just one technique.

Once you know a particular technique well, you can be comfortable not practicing it because you will know that you can call it up at any time; but if you have not studied it at all, you will be tense about your ignorance. Japanese calligraphers need dozens of different brushes for different calligraphic techniques; each morning they prepare all of them so that they are ready whenever they need to use any one of them. It is the same with Ohashiatsu: Study hard so that you are ready to use any technique; get as much information as possible in order to be free *not* to use it. Otherwise, you will forever be a prisoner of what you don't know.

When you start to apply techniques to a receiver, you will find that the receiver's needs will also guide you. Some people have more tension in their necks, some in their backs; some can tolerate a great deal of pressure, others cannot. If you "listen" carefully, the receiver will always let you know which techniques are right for him or her. When you are beginning, try to find the most tolerant receiver you can, so that you are free to develop your rhythm and confidence without worrying too much about causing discomfort.

Then seek out more difficult receivers—they can teach you how tense you are, how you are fighting yourself. You have to challenge yourself or you will not know what your capacity is.

First, practice one technique at a time. Then, learn to make transitions from one technique to another, and then to develop sequences. Each chapter in Part II contains a series of techniques; but again, each of these chapters includes more techniques than you would use in any one session. I show you a full range of possibilities, grouped according to the part of the body being worked on and generally arranged in the sequence I would follow from one part of the body to the next. Out of these longer sequences, you may create your own. You might begin with a leg technique when the receiver is face-up; then, you might practice rotating the leg and getting into position for a different leg technique; then, you might want to practice making a transition from the leg to the arm. In this way, you will eventually design a session—by choosing as many techniques as the receiver can accept and as you have time for, by balancing one with another (by alternating yin and yang meridians, for instance), and by making smooth transitions.

Many factors will influence your choice. Primary among them should be your own position and movement. Avoid awkward transitions that require you to move too great a distance; they can disrupt the flow of a session. You would not want to go from working on the lower leg to working on the neck, for instance. Gradual change is usually best; it makes the receiver feel more secure, and it allows the giver to focus on one technique at a time.

At the beginning of your practice, you must pay special attention to your own body in relation to the receiver. Move as little and as efficiently as possible. You may feel self-conscious at first, but eventually you will move so effortlessly that you will be more conscious of the receiver than of yourself. If you can be free of your own bodywork, you can be free to work on another. Remember: A well-designed Ohashiatsu session should flow as beautifully and naturally as a well-choreographed dance.

Throughout this book, there are photographs in which I demonstrate techniques and sequences for all the basic positions a receiver can comfortably be in. But you will be the one to decide, finally, which positions to use and in which order in any given session. Part III shows you how to move the receiver from one position to another, and it gives some sample sequences, to help you think about creating your own.

This book is designed to be both a workbook and a reference book—come back to it again after you have been practicing Ohashiatsu for a while. By using the table of contents, you can locate a given position for any area of the receiver's body that you wish to work on. At the beginning of each section, there is a list of the techniques to be found in that section. Check your technique against the book. Use the book to evaluate and improve your own bodywork. When you experience any difficulty in your practice (wrist pain, neck pain, or fatigue, for instance) come back to the kata exercises in Chapter 2. The more advanced you become, the more you have to return to the basics. I want this to be a book you will still refer to and appreciate years from now. As you master the techniques presented here, I sincerely hope that each of you will become more flexible, healthier, and happier.

PART I

Principles and Preparation

Always consider yourself an amateur.

Waste your money, but don't waste your time because time never comes back.

CHAPTER

PRINCIPLES

Four main principles distinguish Ohashiatsu from other shiatsu/bodywork methods:

    1. Just be there; don't press.
    2. Use both hands.
    3. Be continuous.
    4. Be natural.

Together these principles determine the movements and techniques of Ohashiatsu, so it is important to understand them before you begin to practice.

PRINCIPLE #1: JUST BE THERE; DON'T PRESS

Be in Tonus

Don't press means don't work, don't maneuver, don't get tired. Ohashiatsu is primarily about *not* doing. Your body has to be in a state of tonus, in which the muscles are relaxed yet ready—and you must maintain this tonicity during the entire treatment. Other shiatsu techniques emphasize where, how, how many times, and how hard to press the receiver, but not what to do with your own body. To practice Ohashiatsu, you must first be in *tonus;* tonus is *being.* The bigger, the heavier, the more difficult the receiver, the more you have to give yourself up to (be in) tonus. This is especially difficult for people who feel they must *do* something—and, therefore, immediately become tense. Ohashiatsu is very good practice for learning how to maintain a calm, meditative, natural body.

In Ohashiatsu, instead of pressing, the giver *leans into* the receiver and the receiver *supports* the giver. Their bodies must be in perfect physiological and spiritual balance. The closer they become, the deeper they connect—just as in every other human relationship. In fact, the proper Ohashiatsu relationship is also expressed in the Japanese character for human.

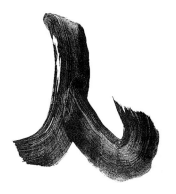

And again, just as we say "human being" rather than "human doing," the Ohashiatsu relationship is one of being, not doing.

The principle of *Don't press* aims at this state of being. If you are *doing*—pressing with your shoulders, arms, or hands—you soon will be tensed up and will exhaust your body. When you press, it is your ego pressing. You sweat, you get tired, you injure your hands and muscles—and you will only be able to give about three treatments a day. But if you stay in tonus as you bring your body to the receiver, without tension, you will actually be stronger and more powerful; you will be able to give better—and more—treatments. Any receiver can tell how relaxed, how meditative you are—the receiver is the mirror of your practice. Ohashiatsu is a form of active, mutual meditation.

Because *shiatsu* comes from *shi* (finger) and *atsu* (pressure), many people believe that you must press particular points. When I studied shiatsu with Japanese teachers, none of them ever said "Don't press." But in Ohashiatsu, you bring your entire body—not just your fingers or hands—to the receiver, and you lean with gravity and tonicity, not with pressure.

Being in tonus is not doing, but being *ready* to do. When I am driving my car on the parkway, I am in tonus. If a deer jumps out in front of my car, I am ready to respond immediately because I am not engaged in anything else and don't have to shift my attention. Race-car drivers are not driving; they are meditating. In Ohashiatsu, when you are in tonus, you can be more aware of your own body movements, your own being. And when you are in this meditative state, you can also be more sensitive to the receiver's health and well-being. Ironically, if you are *doing* (if you are worrying about whether your technique is improving or whether the receiver is getting better) you can-

not fully respond to the receiver's needs and, therefore, your treatment is not as powerful. Many people are so result-oriented that they sabotage their own efforts. Ohashiatsu has such good results because we are not prisoners of the result.

Move from the Hara

Hara means vital center of life; it is the center of *being*, the center of gravity, and the center of all movement and communication in Ohashiatsu. Physically, the hara is the area between the rib cage and the pelvic bone. If you want to increase pressure at any point on the receiver's body, you bring your hara to that point; the shorter the distance between your hara and the receiver, the deeper you go. Don't press with your hand; just move your hara closer to your hand and your entire body will follow. Because your hand isn't pressing, it is free to feel any response from the receiver.

When you move from your hara, your touch is

deeper and more powerful. I am very small, but because I use my hara, I can apply profound pressure without pressing. When you work on a baby or child, you don't need to bring your hara as close as you do to an adult. But however close it is, your hand remains the same—always relaxed—so that you can tell how the receiver is reacting. When the receiver feels pain, the giver's hand starts trembling and tightening.

Ohashiatsu is *Ohara*shiatsu. When you come from your own center, you can connect with the receiver's center. When you bring your entire body to the receiver, you also bring your entire being.

Pull Rather Than Push

Japanese movement (as in sumo and aikido) uses pulling rather than pushing. Ohashiatsu is a pulling technique. *Pushing* means fighting against the receiver; *pulling* means surrendering. When you move toward the receiver from your hara, you follow the force of gravity. You don't push your hara; you are pulled by it. Lower your hara and your whole body will be lowered. You will feel as though you are pulling the receiver's body toward you—that you are being pulled together—not that you are pushing yours toward him. You are using

the receiver's body as well as your own. The bigger the receiver, the bigger your advantage. So if you have a big body, if you are very powerful as a giver, surrender it all and use the receiver's body instead. If you are very small and have little strength, you are lucky; you can give beautiful Ohashiatsu. Ohashiatsu is both for people who have strength and for people who don't, because Ohashiatsu requires effortless movement rather than strength. In Ohashiatsu, pull—don't push.

I want to emphasize this: If you start pressing

with your hand and caring for the receiver first, you cannot give to the receiver. But if you learn to move with your entire body and not just one part, your hands can concentrate on the receiver's response. When you are free of your own body, you are completely dedicated to the receiver.

PRINCIPLE #2: USE BOTH HANDS

In Ohashiatsu you use two hands because humans *have* two hands. Using two hands allows you to be well-balanced as you lean into the receiver. It also allows you to feel with one hand the receiver's reaction to what the other hand is doing. When you use only one hand, you have no other point of reference; you cannot tell what harm you may be doing. When you use only one hand, you cannot have a sense of balance.

When you use two hands, you will also find that you can support your own body more easily and move around the receiver with less effort. Because you will be less tired, you will be able to give more treatments—and not just more treatments in a single day; you also will be able to give treatments for many more years if you take care to work safely and naturally—with *two* hands. When you move in a simple and balanced way, Ohashiatsu becomes a beautiful, enjoyable dance.

Meridian Lines

Many bodywork methods, especially shiatsu, emphasize putting pressure—often with just one finger—on single points, or *tsubos*. Sometimes they call for the use of two hands, but usually with one hand on top of the other and still pressing on only one point. This can be extremely uncomfortable—even painful—for both the giver and the receiver. Ohashiatsu does not focus on points but works with two hands along the *meridian lines,* the pathways of energy in the body.

Using two hands on two different points of a meridian enables you to follow the meridian line more easily, to concentrate on certain places more than others, and to increase the chance of reaching those places where the receiver may wish to have longer, deeper, or even stronger touch or treat-ment. And in the end, because they lie along the meridian lines, you are also satisfying tsubo needs.

Because Ohashiatsu uses two hands on meridian lines, not one finger on one point, it never causes unnecessary pain, although you may be applying the same amount of pressure as you would with one hand. The second hand creates a distraction that diverts the receiver's attention and allows him or her to relax and open up. Some people don't believe I am leaning deeply enough when they feel no pain. They ask me, "Ohashi, are you pressing? I don't feel any pain." So I release one hand slowly, and then they feel the pain and real-ize I am working deeply. We are funny about pain: If there is none, we don't believe we are being stimulated.

Mother Hand and Messenger Hand

When you use two hands in Ohashiatsu, one hand is called the *mother* hand, the other the *messenger* hand. The mother hand, which doesn't move, diagnoses and communicates with the receiver; the messenger hand then applies pressure accordingly. You will use the bigger, fleshier areas—such as the palm—of the mother hand, and you will use the smaller, bonier areas—such as the thumb and knuckle—of the messenger hand.

Ohashiatsu is a mother-hand technique: The messenger hand is directed and controlled by the mother hand. Other shiatsu methods are messenger-hand-oriented. Yes, we need the messenger hand's work, but the mother hand is actually far more important. Note carefully in the photographs of this book the location of my mother hand and how I use it—it is essential.

Diagnosis

In Ohashiatsu, it is important to be diagnosing at every moment: where the receiver has pain and how much; where to apply pressure, how much pressure to apply, and for how long. The mother hand can tell whether the receiver is improving and whether the treatment is working. As in other Oriental practices, in Ohashiatsu every moment of treatment is also diagnosis, thanks to the mother hand.

You may be asking yourself if this focus on the receiver conflicts with our precept that Ohashiatsu is for givers. It does not. When you improve your technique for your own sake, you also improve your powers of diagnosis and treatment. When you improve the result for the receiver, you also benefit yourself.

PRINCIPLE #3: BE CONTINUOUS

I designed Ohashiatsu to be like a stream of water, flowing seamlessly from beginning to end. Once you put your hands on the receiver, you keep your hands on until the session is finished. Continuity of movement helps the receiver to relax and maintain trust at all times because he or she always knows where the giver is and where the giver is going. When I touch a horse, for example, I go first to the nose, then to the neck, torso, and flanks. The horse never gets nervous, because he knows where I am going. Continuity means no surprises. If you lean into one point, and then remove your hands and lean into another, the receiver is surprised, becomes guarded and defensive, and the giver cannot go deeper. When you maintain continuous contact, the receiver can relax and surrender to the treatment.

Continuity also means following the meridian

lines. If you work only the tsubo points, one and then the next, you will lose touch with the receiver. But a meridian line is continuous. You move from one part of a meridian to the next part of that meridian, from one meridian to the next meridian, and from one part of the body to the next part of the body. When you change the receiver's position—say, from face-up to face-down—you must also practice continuity.

When my movements are continuous, they become so effortless that my body seems to disappear. And once my body disappears, I can give a wonderful treatment. Remember: I don't *give* Ohashiatsu, I *become* Ohashiatsu. I am not *doing*, I am *being*. And when I am being, no matter how big the receivers' bodies are, they shrink and shrink and suddenly they, too, disappear; they are being with me: Receiver and giver are one, which is the ultimate goal. When treatment is complete, suddenly my body comes back, and then the receiver's body comes back. "Oh, my goodness!" I say. "I didn't know you were still here!" They say, "Oh, my goodness, Ohashi! I didn't know you were still here!" We had both disappeared because continuity allowed us to do so.

PRINCIPLE #4: BE NATURAL

It is fashionable nowadays in many bodywork methods to talk about whether or not givers have sufficient *ki* (vital energy). Some emphasize ki almost relentlessly, but doing so will only bring suffering to both the giver and the receiver. If the receiver doesn't feel the giver's ki, the giver will feel inadequate. And if the receiver does feel it, the giver will worry about whether he will have it the next time. Either way, you become a prisoner of ki.

Whether you have ki or not, you must first enjoy what you are doing. If you enjoy, then ki will come to you. And if it should naturally fade, don't despair; sooner or later, if you are open to it, ki will return. You will sense it. But don't pretend to be other than you are. Allow the natural energy to come to you rather than seek it. Become a vessel and allow yourself to be filled.

Don't allow yourself to become attached to the notion of ki. You are only an instrument; recognize that healing is not in your own hands. Don't accept compliments; once you start taking credit, deterioration and downfall are not far behind. *Being natural* also means being compassionate. Feel healing love toward the receiver. Believe in the universal higher energy.

Cross-Patterning

When we are babies, one of our first movements is pushing ourselves up from a prone position with our hands. We call this kind of movement *homologous*—movement of the two upper limbs or two lower limbs at the same time and in the same direction. During this movement, we are developing flexibility in our cervical vertebrae (our newborn spines are straight). Homologous movement is very strenuous and we cannot do it for very long. As adults we don't do much of it other than lifting (for instance, lifting heavy dumbbells over our heads).

At about three or four months of age, babies start turning to their right and left sides. We call this *homolateral* movement (*lateral* means side). Again, as adults we don't experience much homolateral movement (except, for instance, in fencing and some dancing—but you cannot dance homolaterally for long).

Next, babies start crawling and their bodies develop the cervical, thoracic, and lumbar vertebrae in preparation for standing up. This crawling process is *cross-patterning* movement, meaning that you move your right hand and left knee, or left hand and right knee (one hand and the opposite knee) simultaneously. Ninety-nine percent of our movement is cross-patterning: walking, running, dancing, skating, cross-country skiing. Cross-patterning gives us maximum balance for the least effort. Less effort means less fatigue, and that means you can continue longer. Cross-patterning is our most natural movement.

Some shiatsu practitioners emphasize homologous movement: They apply their thumbs and press back and forth. This is painful for the receiver and can eventually result in lower back pain for the giver. Another common form of shiatsu employs homolateral movement, in which the right hand and right knee move together. Again, this method can be painful to both giver and receiver. In Ohashiatsu cross-patterning, however,

you use your entire body, much as a baby does when it crawls. You move your right hand two inches and, simultaneously, you move your left knee two inches; your entire body follows your hands. When you use two hands and cross-patterning, your body moves not in a series of abrupt zigzag movements but in a continuous figure 8. As long as you move your body naturally and continuously , you can give five to ten treatments a day. In the illustrations throughout this book, pay close attention to how the movements of my hands and knees (and even my toes) are coordinated: If I move my right thumb, for example, I also move my left big toe. Only in cross-patterning does the entire body participate, and cross-patterning is the basic movement of Ohashiatsu. There are exercises to help you master this movement in Chapter 2.

1. Just be there; don't press.
2. Use both hands.
3. Be continuous.
4. Be natural.

If you always keep these four principles in mind, you will find that your practice of Ohashiatsu will become effortless and artful. Indeed, when you master an art, you no longer practice it: I don't practice Ohashiatsu; I become it. I don't *do*; I *am*. If you are what you are doing, you are free from what you are doing. This is the goal you should aim for as you follow the exercises and techniques presented in this book.

TABLE 1

DIFFERENCES BETWEEN OHASHIATSU AND SHIATSU

OHASHIATSU	SHIATSU
Attitude: Holistic	Attitude: Symptomatic
Giver's body: Tonus	Giver's body: Tense
Don't press	Press hard
Pull	Press, push
Hara, whole body	Finger pressure, muscle power
Body-mind: Psychological, spiritual	Body: Physical
Benefit for giver and receiver	Benefit for receiver
Continuous movement	Abrupt movement
Giver meditates	Giver works hard
Cross-patterning	Homologous, homolateral
Meridians	Points
Two hands, two points	One point
Comfortably deep	Painful
Caring and supporting	Preoccupied, busy
Bodywork for giver	Bodywork for receiver

CHAPTER

Kata:

Form and

Movement

In any activity in which movement is important (dancing, martial arts, cooking, flower arranging, performing the tea ceremony, even driving a car) there are basic forms that dictate the patterns to be followed. Without mastering the basic movements (in Japanese the term is *kata*), we cannot go on to more advanced movements or techniques. Whenever we experience difficulty learning more advanced or more complicated techniques—whenever we experience pain or injury, whenever our body forgets how to move—we have to return to the basic movements.

When I was a novice, I liked to show off, to use techniques that I thought would impress. Now, after years of experience and study, I have happily returned to basic movements that allow my body to work more efficiently and to produce better results. These movements look effortless, like those of a beginner. What a wonderful metamorphosis—becoming a beginner again!

This chapter presents the basic forms and movements of Ohashiatsu, as well as exercises (some to do alone and some to do with a partner) that will prepare you for their use in an actual session.

In the 1970s I gave some sessions to the late prima ballerina Margot Fonteyn. After one of them, she said she was attending ballet classes for beginners. I asked her, "Why are you—a famous, top ballerina—taking a beginner's basic course, with 18-year-old kids?" She said, "If I don't take this class every day, I can tell it in my performance; and if I don't take this class for two days, my choreographer can tell; and if I don't take it for three days, an experienced audience can tell." Even after more than 20 years of dancing, Margot Fonteyn practiced the basic movements of ballet technique in order to maintain her extraordinary performances on stage.

SUPPORTING

Supporting may seem to be neither a form nor a movement. Actually, it is something of both and it is at the very heart of the relationship between giver and receiver in Ohashiatsu, which is a relationship of mutual trust. To support in the right way means to appreciate your physical, mental, and spiritual being, to be aware of the universe, to *be* with yourself and your partner. It is a relationship of *being*, not doing. And yet, each partner depends on the other; neither could maintain his or her position without the other. So, in a way, supporting *is* a kind of doing—it is where activity and passivity come together.

The following exercises are to help you learn how to be in tonus when you support and are supported. First you practice alone—against a wall and on a scale. Then you practice with a partner.

Leaning against a wall

Practice this technique in order to cultivate your sense of tonus. Put either your elbow or palm against a wall, and lean. As you lean, surrender yourself to the wall. You must trust that the wall will not fall without warning. When you do this, you will find that the wall welcomes your body weight; it will feel almost as though the wall were coming towards you. Your entire body, including your toes, fingers, shoulders, back, and neck, should be relaxed and in a state of tonus.

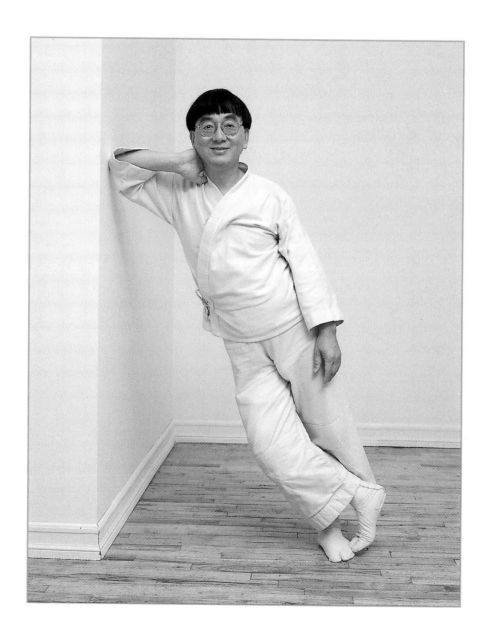

Leaning on a bathroom scale

Kneel down on the floor next to a bathroom scale and place both hands on it. Press the scale as hard as you can. (You may sweat and grunt, if you like.) Remember the number that registers on the scale when you press your hardest.

Next, keep your hands on the scale and move your knees further back, into a crawling position, with your upper legs at about a 90-degree angle to your torso. Straighten your arms and spine, which will widen the angle. Lean on the scale by bringing the center of your body, your hara, closer to the scale (we call this "leaning from your hara"). Keep your entire body relaxed, and smile. Now look at the number that registers. You'll be surprised to see that the more you relax and remain in tonus (the more you engage your hara) the heavier you will become. Now you can see why it is unwise to press: When you are holding your body in tonus, gravity alone will bring you to the receiver. The meridians and tsubos are waiting for you.

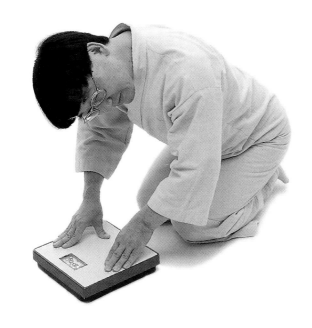

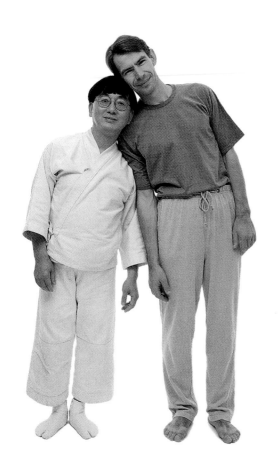

Leaning side by side

When two human beings touch, just by *being* they start doing.

Stand side by side and lean against your partner, so that you are supporting each other's shoulders and heads but also relaxing completely. Neither of you is *doing* anything, but without each other you could not maintain this position; you are both *supporting*. In Ohashiatsu, no one is exclusively either a giver or a receiver; as in life, we support each other. Neither of us can stand alone.

Leaning back to back

Place your back against that of your partner. The more you and he trust each other in this position, the more comfortable and peaceful you will be. When you surrender to your partner, you leave your entire safety to him; in the process, you also become sensitive to his condition. This is a principle of Oriental diagnosis: you don't look for problems; you trust the receiver to show you what is imbalanced or uncomfortable.

Now, suppose the two of you started pushing against each other, grunting and sweating and tensing your muscles. Within minutes, both of you would be tired and frustrated and in danger of falling over. (Note that the basic posture would *look* the same, whether you are in a relaxed state—tonus—or in a tense state.) So remember always to be in tonus. Be there; don't press.

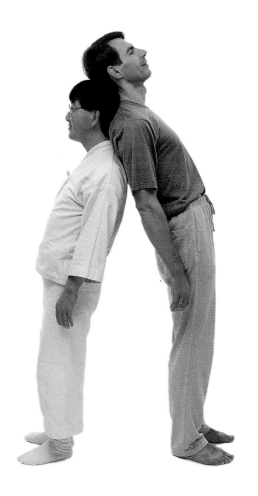

Standing and kneeling

In this kata, you kneel with your arms raised and your palms spread. Your partner stands facing away from you and leans back onto your waiting hands. The more he trusts, the more he will lean, and the more important will be the support you give him. (Also, as he leans into your hands, he will feel deep, comfortable pressure.) If you push rather than support, you can lose your importance by pushing your partner too far; that is, into an upright position, where he does not need any support.

Next, switch places with your partner and repeat the exercise.

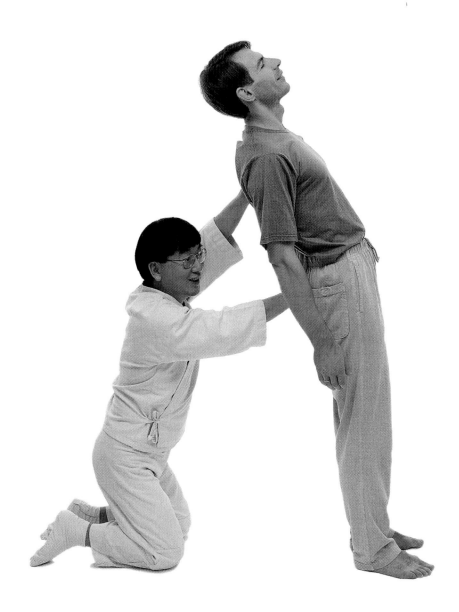

Sitting down and standing up

Stand 2 to 3 feet behind your partner, who sits on the floor with his legs outstretched. Lean forward and place your hands on his shoulders as he leans back toward you. Your arms should make a straight line with his torso.

In this position, both of you are supporting each other equally: One of you would fall forward and the other would fall backward if each were not there; you are in tonus.

Switch positions with your partner and repeat.

Your relationship with your partner in this kata can be imagined as the side legs of an equilateral triangle, where the giver and the receiver are mutually dependent—just as in all healthy human relationships. In fact, this position resembles the Japanese character for *human*:

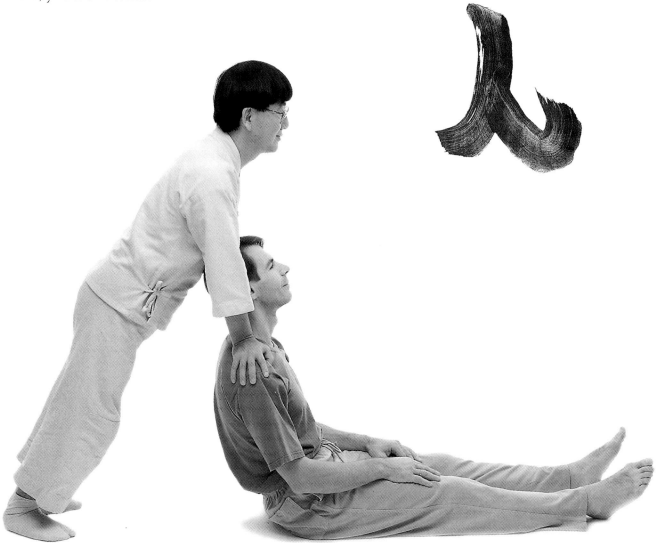

CRAWLING

Crawling is a very important kata in Ohashiatsu, and it is a good form of bodywork in itself. When you crawl, you move a hand and the opposite knee at the same time; you coordinate the right and left sides of your body along a diagonal axis. This form of movement is called cross-patterning. Notice that it is impossible to crawl if you try to move all your hands and knees at once, or just both hands or both knees. We always move one hand and the opposite knee at the same time because that keeps our balance and is effortless and comfortable. Cross-patterning is the most common form of movement in our daily lives, and it can make you a most efficient bodyworker.

In Ohashiatsu, one hand and the opposite knee move together as you work along a meridian. I call these the *messenger hand* and the *messenger knee*. The hand and knee that remain stationary are the *mother hand* and *mother knee*. (These will be discussed in more detail later.) Pay more attention to your knees than to your hands when you are crawling, to increase your awareness of your entire body movement.

The word *manipulation*, which comes from the Latin term for *handful*, is often used in bodywork and physical therapies. The word *shiatsu*, which translates as *finger pressure*, also emphasizes the hand. Some bodyworkers think their arms and hands are the most important part of their anatomy for their job. But in Ohashiatsu, the entire body works in balanced, effortless harmony, as it does when we crawl. The entire body becomes our hand.

I recommend even to my advanced students that they crawl for several minutes before they practice Ohashiatsu. Whenever you feel confused in your technique, practice crawling.

Crawling alone

In a crawling position, space your hands and knees on the floor equally far apart and perpendicular to your torso. Relax your back muscles, fingers, and toes. Move your left hand forward 5 inches and notice that you will also (almost involuntarily) move your right knee forward 5 inches in order to keep your balance. Continue to crawl around the room until the movement feels thoroughly natural. You will discover that the crawling position is extremely comfortable. I have found that crawling is especially good for the prevention and treatment of lower back pain and sciatica.

The cross-patterning movement that charac-terizes crawling also encourages brain development and coordination. Some institutions that care for the mentally handicapped teach crawling. I tell my students that the more they crawl, the smarter they will become.

You may discover other benefits of crawling. When you get up in the morning, try crawling out from your bed and crawling around your room to the bathroom. You may be surprised to discover loose change on your floor as well as rings, earrings, keys, and buttons you lost ages ago. Ohashiatsu can make you richer and your room cleaner, too!

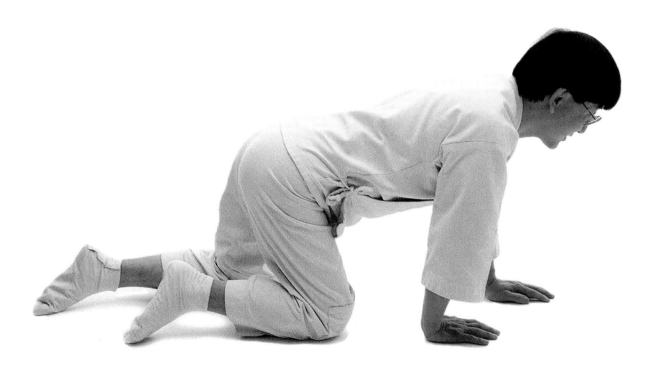

Moving your hara in the crawling position

After crawling, stay in position with your palms flat on the floor. Close your eyes and move your hara in the pattern of a figure 8. You will notice that you are shifting your body weight to four different points.

You will use this figure 8 movement almost continuously during an Ohashiatsu session as you shift your weight from mother hand and knee to messenger hand and knee.

If you can, get four bath scales and place each of your hands and knees on one of the scales to measure how your weight shifts during this kata.

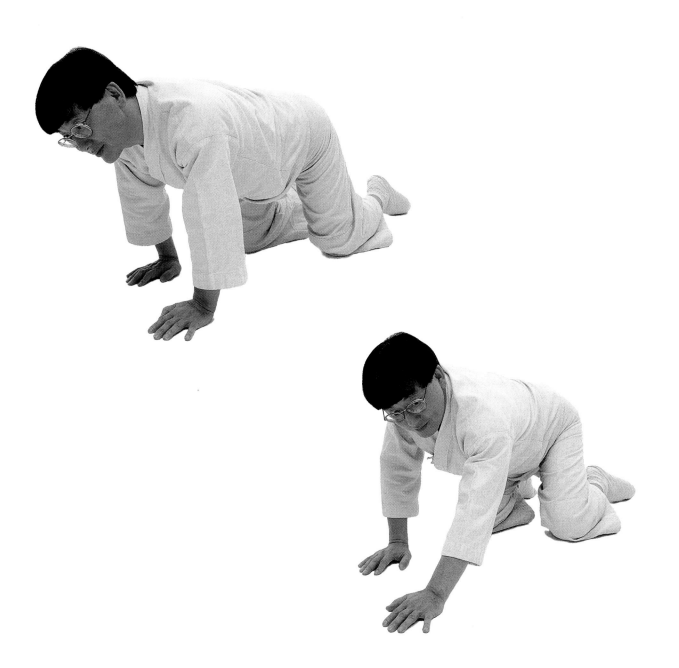

Moving your hara in the crawling position with a partner

Get a partner and face him in the crawling position. Place your left shoulder against his left shoulder, and start moving your hara in harmony with his. When he moves forward, you move backward; when he moves to the side, you follow—and so on, in a figure 8 pattern. Don't change the position of your hands or knees. Continue until the two of you are moving effortlessly together.

Synchronize your breathing; harmonize your movement without talking to each other. Sense each other's movement . . . don't resist or fight; accept each other . . . don't lose each other.

Next, try placing an orange or apple between your shoulders while you practice the figure 8 pattern. Don't crush or drop it. If you accomplish this feat, congratulate yourselves!

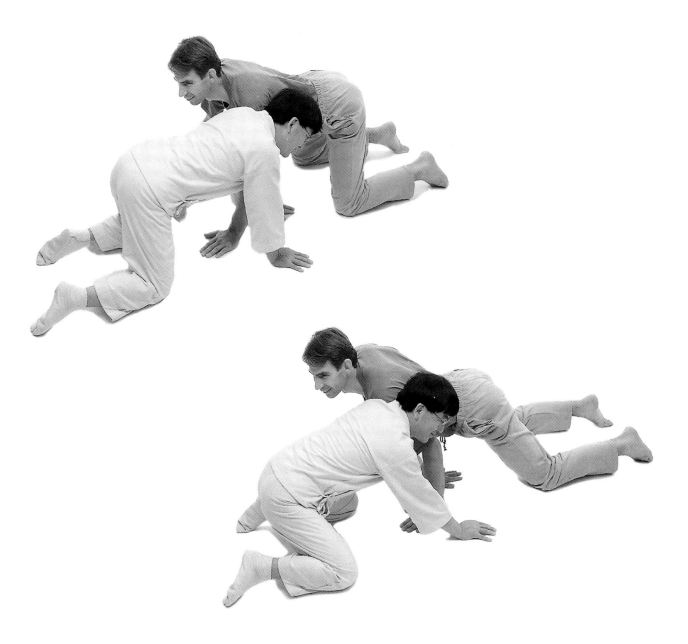

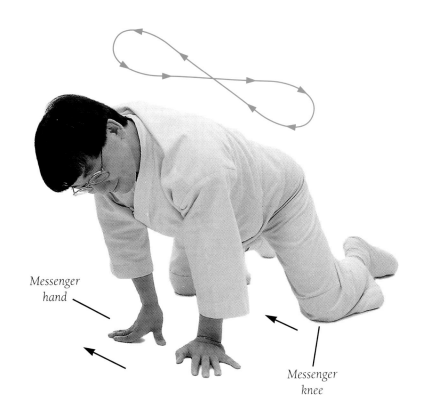

Messenger
hand

Messenger
knee

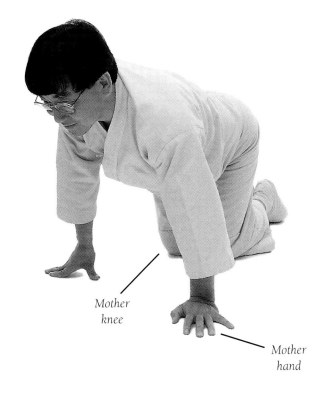

Mother
knee

Mother
hand

Hand technique in the crawling position

Put your left hand flat on the floor; put your right hand down with only the thumb and fingers touching the floor. Consider your left hand your mother hand and the opposite knee (the right) your mother knee. Your right hand is the messenger hand, and your left knee is the messenger knee. Next, move your hara in a figure 8 pattern. Lean into your thumb and hold; then release pressure and move your thumb about 3 inches to the right, as though you were pressing along a meridian line. When you move your right hand, move your left (messenger) knee the same distance; your mother hand and mother knee remain stationary. Don't tense any muscles; make sure your toes are not curled under or up (we sometimes do this unconsciously).

When your left knee reaches your right knee, let your left hand become the messenger hand and your right knee the messenger knee. Then continue in the *same direction* until your left hand reaches your right hand.

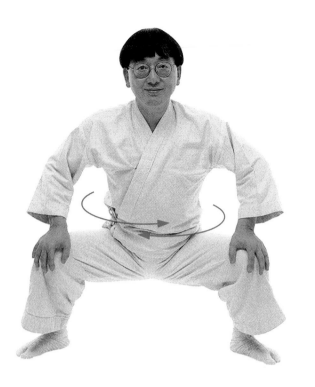

LOWERING YOUR HARA

Shiko exercise

This exercise, like the next two, helps to open the hip socket and lower your hara. The objective of the first part of the exercise is to shift your body weight as low as possible.

Stand with your spine straight and arms down. Now open your legs as wide as you comfortably can. Place your hands, palms down, on your knees, and bend your knees. Start moving your hara slowly in a circle, first clockwise, then counterclockwise.

Now, raise one leg and stretch it out to the side. Then bring your foot down to the floor and lower your hips as far as possible. Move from side to side slowly several times. Feel your hip sockets opening.

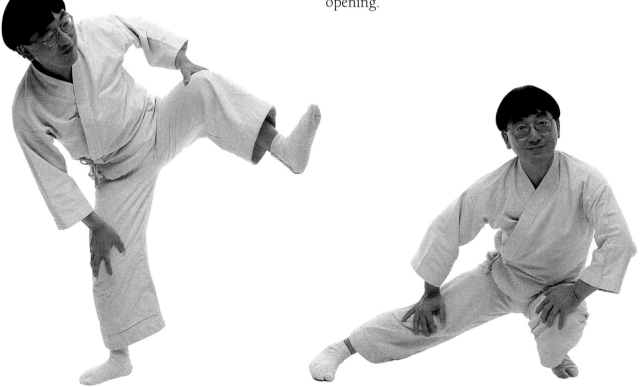

Now, repeat with the other leg.

After this warm-up routine, return to a standing position with your knees bent and your feet as close together as possible. Next, lift your left leg as high as you can, first in front of you and then to the side. Now, bring your foot down quickly, as though you were slapping the floor. Call out "Ki-ai!" in a loud, deep voice. It will energize and inspire you.

Repeat with the right leg and then continue, alternating legs, for as long as you can.

Note: Do this sequence with caution. Don't overstretch; be sure your movements are slow. If you feel any pain or difficulty, stand up and walk around the room; rotate your knees gently.

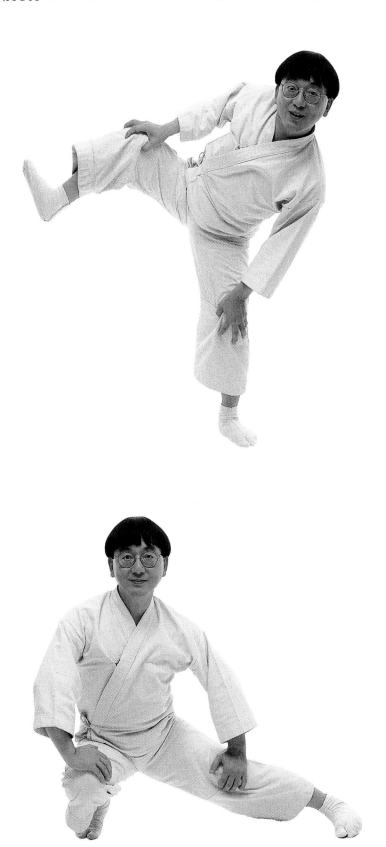

The shiko exercise is an important kata for Japanese martial arts, especially sumo wrestling. A champion of the sumo tournament is called yokozuna. The first and current champion is a Hawaiian named Akebono. When he came to Japan, he had to practice this shiko exercise 400 times every morning in order to lower his gravity before he was allowed to have breakfast. Because he was a dedicated apprentice, he lowered his hara enough to kick Japanese wrestlers out of the ring!

Lowering your hara in a figure 8

This exercise is to help you learn to raise and lower your hara as you move in the figure 8 pattern.

Stand straight with your feet parallel; relax your entire body. You should feel not so much that you are standing as that the floor is supporting you. The top of your head, neck, spine, knees, and ankles should be in a line. You may want to close your eyes.

Next, imagine that you are a wondrous tube connecting heaven and earth, receiving heaven's energy from above and earth's energy from below. Bring both hands in front of your chest with palms outward; bend your knees slightly. Don't tense

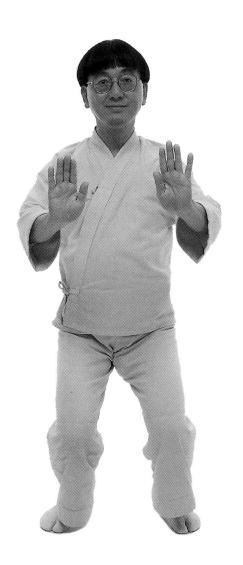

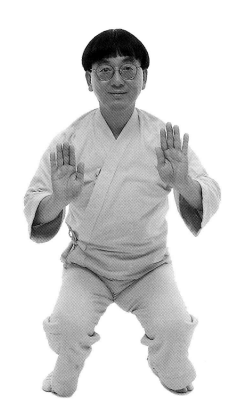

anything. Now, without moving your feet, move your hara to the left and notice that your hands and knees also move to the left. Even though you did not intentionally move them, they moved because your hara moved. Now, bring your hara back to the center. Your hands and knees will follow. Repeat to the right side and then back to center. Now bend your knees more and move your hara down. Move up again. Now, combine these up and down and left to right movements in a

smooth pattern to make a figure 8. Note that your hands are moving even though you don't intend to move them; your intention is in your hara.

Next, begin to enlarge the figure 8 and allow your arms to move in a figure 8 pattern too. This is a t'ai chi movement. Ohashiatsu is like a t'ai chi exercise on the floor. You will use this movement as you work on certain parts of the body (when you rotate the legs, for instance, or stretch the neck).

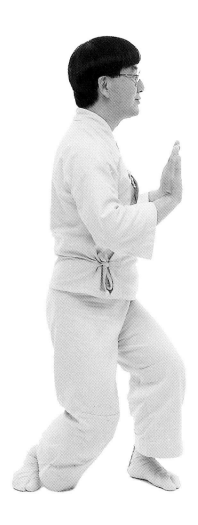
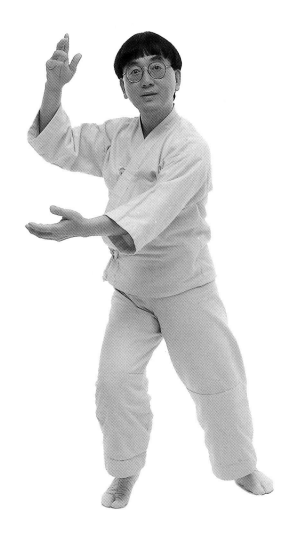

Pulling down to lower your hara

You will use this movement when you are working on the meridians in the leg and neck areas.

Kneel down on your right knee; keep your left knee raised with the foot flat on the floor. Cross your arms with your palms down. Move your hips up and down, raising and lowering your hands as you do so. (Your feet should remain as they were.) You should have the sense that you are *pulling* your hara toward the floor; your hands, being guided by your hara, will also move down as you do this. As your legs become more flexible, you will be able to go lower and lower.

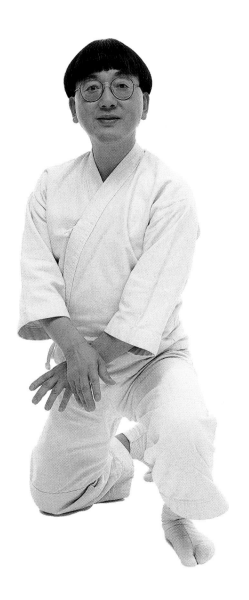
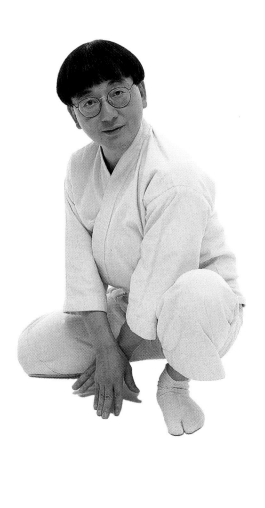

SQUATTING

Squatting with a straight spine

This exercise is primarily to prepare you for maintaining balance and flexibility while working on a small area, such as the neck.

Stand with your feet parallel, your spine straight, and your body relaxed. Lower your hara by slowly bending your knees. Keep your spine straight; your knees can be together or apart. Once you are in a squatting position, notice that your toes (especially the big toes) are supporting your straight back. Next, slowly place your right knee on the floor. In order to keep a straight spine, you will need to shift your right shoulder forward slightly. If you have trouble keeping your balance, raise your left arm in front of you. Now, repeat with the left knee. Always keep a straight spine.

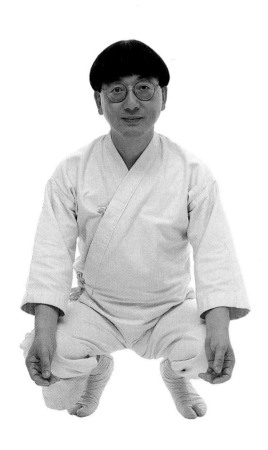

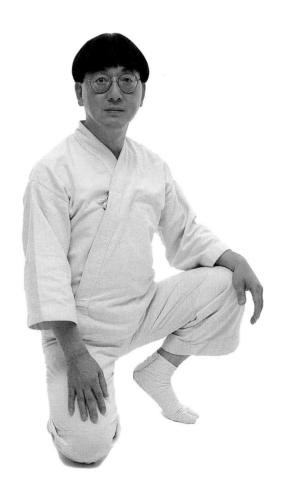

Squat, moving forward with cross-patterning

In this exercise, you move forward in a squatting position.

Squat with your heels raised. Place your right knee on the floor and bring your left arm forward. Now switch your knees and your arms. Do this two or three times, alternating legs. Now, coordinate your arms with your legs by rotating the opposite arm over your head as each leg comes forward (right arm with left leg, and so on). Do this exercise as if you were a quietly turning wheel.

Next, begin to move in a straight line for about 30 feet (if you have the space); turn around while still squatting and go in the opposite direction. Keep your spine straight and your shoulders relaxed. Don't make a noise when your knees touch the floor. Don't sweat! You'll notice that your hip socket is opening more and your big toe is getting more flexible. These are desirable changes for practicing Ohashiatsu.

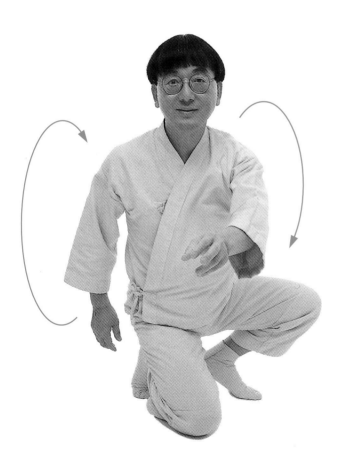 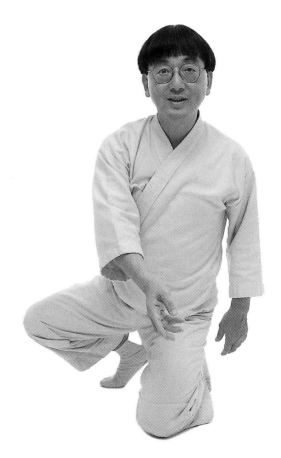

Squat, moving side to side

This exercise will help increase your flexibility and stability.

Keep your spine straight and squat down with your heels raised. Raise your arms in front of you, with your palms either up or down. Next, turn to your right, lower your left knee and your right arm. Return to center; then turn to your left, switching knee and arm positions. Continue for as long as you comfortably can.

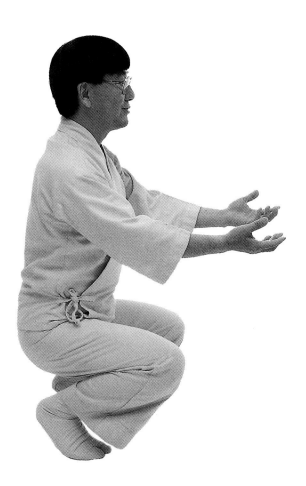

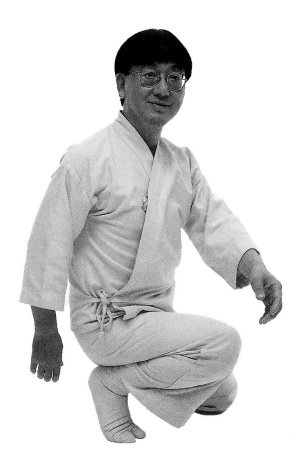

WATCH YOUR BIG TOES

As you are discovering, your big toes are important in keeping your spine straight and your body in balance. A stiff and tight big toe will prevent you from moving easily. When I wake up in the morning, I rotate my toes to examine their flexibility, which helps me to determine how many sessions I am going to give that day. If my toes are tight, my body will tire easily.

I always correct students' hand movements by watching them from the back. When I see their toes, I can see if they are using their hands correctly. Relaxed toes mean relaxed hands and torso.

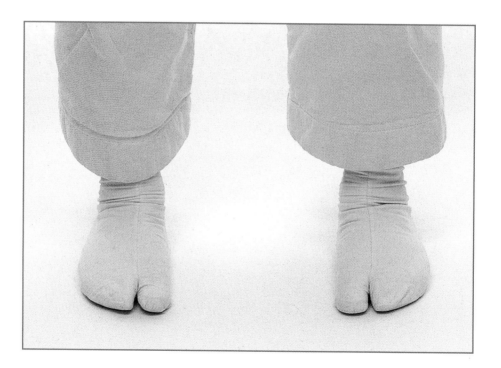

As you can see in this close-up, I wear special Japanese footgear called tabis. They separate the big toes from the other toes, which gives me greater flexibility and balance, so that I can more easily maintain tonus in my body and avoid fatigue. (If you cannot find tabis, you can still probably find socks that separate the toes.)

PART II

The Ohashiatsu
Session

◆

*The body is the physical
manifestation of the soul.*

CHAPTER

3

MOVING IN TONUS . . . THE FACE-UP AND FACE-DOWN POSITIONS

FACE-UP

After you have practiced the kata so often that the basic positions and movements feel completely natural to you, you will be ready to practice them on a receiver. Part II contains techniques for working on various parts of the body when the receiver is in each of the basic Ohashiatsu positions. Here, you will apply what you have learned about supporting and being supported, about moving from your hara, about maintaining balance and continuity, to another person.

Start simply. First, get comfortable bringing your body weight to the receiver; practice the gradual application of pressure from one hand to the other before you try to work along a meridian. When you do work along a meridian, go slowly enough to keep your balance and remember cross-patterning. Don't be afraid to ask the receiver how he or she is reacting.

As you gain confidence, you will begin to move more easily and you will move not just along a meridian on one part of the body but from one part of the body to another. But as you gain confi-

dence and experience, also continue to keep the kata in mind, continue to practice them on your own. They are the foundation of Ohashiatsu—the basic steps that you will now combine into a beautiful choreography of techniques.

Generally speaking, I start an Ohashiatsu session with the receiver in a face-up position. This position is the most effective one for assessing the receiver's condition because it gives me direct access to the hara. But it is also a position that exposes the most sensitive and vulnerable parts of the body. Many people (especially those who don't know me or who have never had Ohashiatsu before) feel uncomfortable beginning in this position. Westerners may not be acquainted with the concept of hara, and even a big, confident receiver might be intimidated by having someone sit above him and touch his stomach. So I don't usually take clients unless they have been referred by someone I have worked with before and know what to expect. If a receiver is new or seems ill at ease, you can begin with another position.

DIAGNOSING THE HARA

Sequence

- ◆ Gasho and meditation
  - Extended arms exercise
  - Initiating the touch
- ◆ The hara
  - Both palms on the hara
  - Fingers on the hara
- ◆ Returning to the hara

The hara is the area of the torso between the solar plexus and the pubic bone. It is more or less a horizontal oval shape, with the rib cage above and the hip bones below.

That is a strictly physical definition. From a Japanese point of view, the hara expresses a person's life energy, dignity, spiritual being, and personality. Since the hara is also a person's center of gravity, it is considered the fulcrum about which any expressive movement must revolve.

The hara is also the diagnostic area of 12 meridians, so we place our hands there first in order to feel what is happening with the receiver's energy flow.

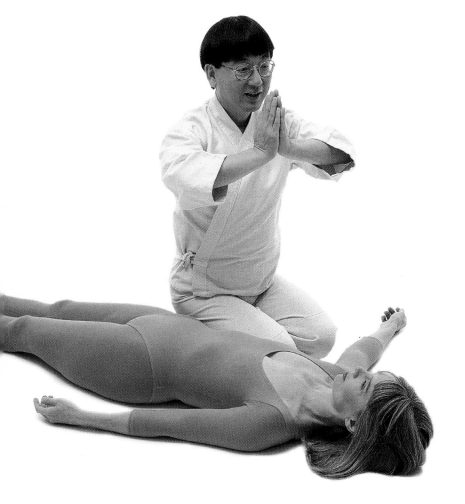

Gasho and meditation

Before I apply my hands to a receiver, I sit in a *seiza* position with my spine straight, elbows raised and bent, with my palms together. I sit as close as possible to the receiver without pressing into her hip bone. Our bodies touch lightly; my shoulders, arms, and fingers are relaxed.

In this position, I concentrate on where and who I am, breathing slowly from the top of my head to the tips of my toes and focusing my sense of being in my hara. Once I sit down in front of the receiver, I am completely detached from any other commitment or activity in my life. I am totally focused on the present moment of *being*. My past, present, and future are all here and now.

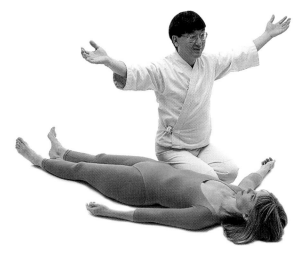

I then stretch out my arms to the sides, bring them above my head, place my palms together, and hold them there for about seven seconds. Slowly, I lower my palms to a position above my heart with both elbows raised horizontally. I then bow three times. In Japanese, we call this action *gasho*. The first bow represents respect to the receiver; the second shows respect to myself; the third shows respect to the higher being. This gasho purifies my intention, focuses my effort, and unifies my body, mind, and spirit.

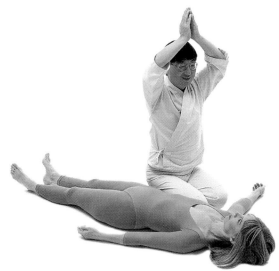

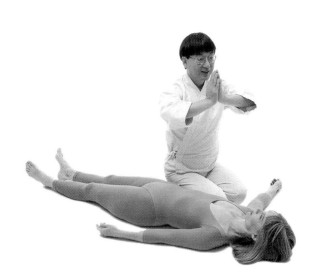

RUBBING DOWN YOUR HANDS

Sometimes before a session I vigorously rub down my hands to bring them more circulation, ki, and concentration. Nobody likes to be touched with cold hands, so rubbing down may be essential unless you have excellent circulation. Fortunately, in Ohashiatsu, the receiver does not need to undress, so he or she may not notice if your hands are cold. During a treatment, your hands will warm up naturally.

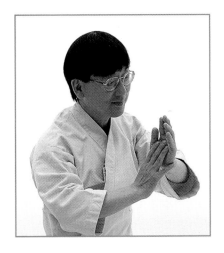

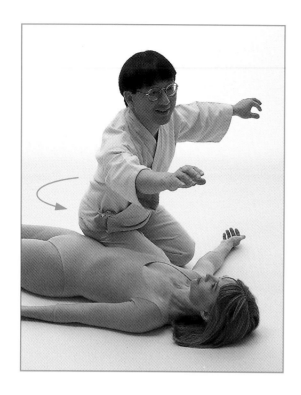

Extended arms exercise

Try this exercise before you put your hands on a receiver's body.

Keep both arms extended in the air; while keeping your spine straight, bring your own hara toward her hara. Next, move your upper body (focusing on your hara at the center) in a figure 8 motion, keeping your arms raised. Repeat the figure 8 three times. Lean into the extreme points of the figure 8; feel the pull of gravity on your torso. You should have the sensation that you may fall if you don't keep moving. Your hands are not so important; your hara movement is more important. Your arms and hands are not *doing*; that is, you are not moving from your arms and hands. When you move from your hara, you can keep your hands relaxed, in a tonus state, enabling you to "listen" more clearly to the receiver's hara.

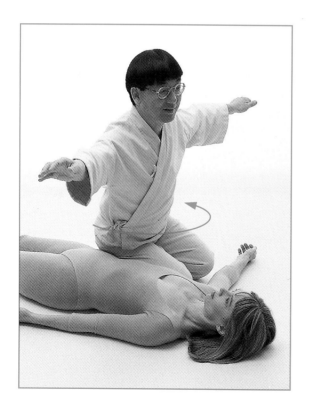

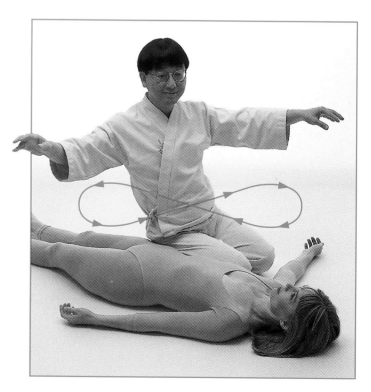

Initiating the touch

You are at last ready to apply your hands to the receiver.

Sit in a seiza position parallel to her right side, and apply your left palm to her forehead and your right palm to her hara, just below the navel. Pick up on her breathing pattern and synchronize your own with it. As she exhales, you exhale and lean toward her from your hara. Once you are breathing together, slowly extend your exhaling and leaning, and she will respond with slower, deeper breaths. Lean and breathe at least three times (or as many as seven, if her breathing is shallow and short).

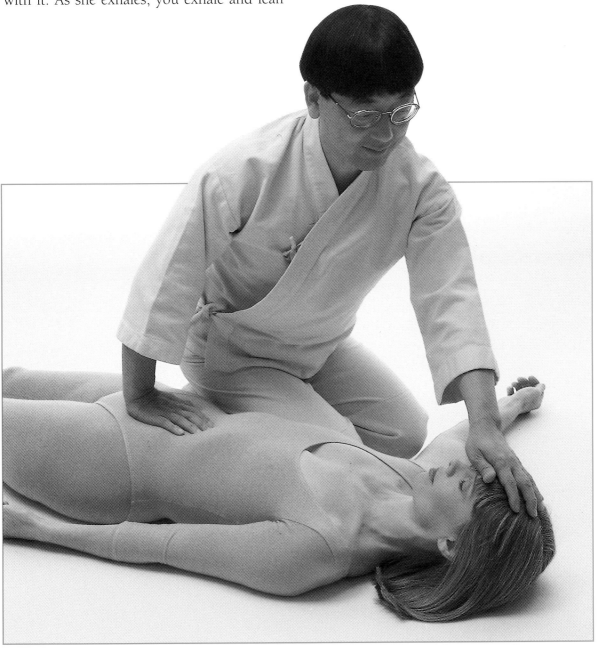

THE HARA

The Hara diagram below shows the area of the hara that corresponds to 12 of the 14 meridians. When you place your hand on these areas, you can feel the general condition of the meridian as well as the amount of energy that has collected at that point. Some areas—where there is a lack of energy—may feel loose; other areas—where there is an excess of energy—may feel tight. The information you gather from touching the hara can guide you as you work on the rest of the body, telling you where and how energy may need to be redistributed in order to restore balance.

Remember that the hara is a very sensitive and vulnerable area. The way you feel when you touch a receiver can determine the way he or she will respond. To encourage the receiver to relax and trust you, you must be relaxed—in tonus—yourself. Try to release any tension from your mind and body. Your touch should be warm and gentle. While your messenger hand explores, your mother hand should soothe and comfort. The connection you establish with your hands can provide an experience of deep communion for both you and the receiver.

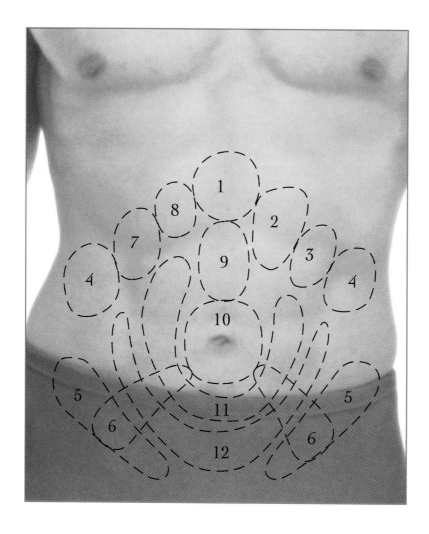

Meridian
Diagnostic Areas

1	Heart
2	Stomach
3	Triple Heater
4	Lung
5	Large Intestine
6	Small Intestine
7	Liver
8	Gall Bladder
9	Heart Constrictor
10	Spleen
11	Kidney
12	Bladder

Both palms on the hara

When your breathing is fully synchronized with that of the receiver, move your left hand (the mother hand) to the area just above the navel in the area associated with the Gall Bladder and Liver meridians; your hand should be open and relaxed with the fingers together. Next, apply your right hand (the messenger hand) just under the solar plexus in the area associated with the Heart meridian (see the Hara chart opposite).

Keep your navel aligned with hers; bring your hara toward hers. The closer your two haras are, the closer and deeper your hands can go (and yet not cause pain to the receiver). Maintain tonus so that you can feel how she is responding to your touch. Your hands and arms will become channels, transmitting her responses to your hara. This process is the true meaning of *setsushin* (touching diagnosis). You are touching her physical body in order to understand her physical, spiritual, and psychic health.

Move your hara first toward your mother hand, then toward your messenger hand. Stay there about two seconds; then lean again toward your mother hand, using a little more body weight; lean again toward the messenger hand, and so on, gradually increasing your body weight

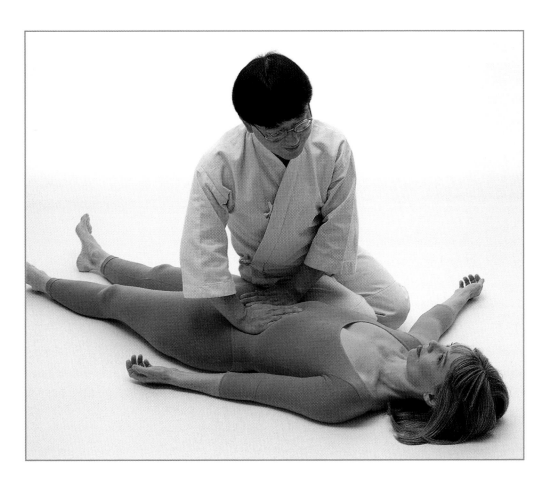

Leaning from your hara

as you go. Shift your weight between your mother hand and messenger hand by moving in a figure 8 pattern, *not* by moving side to side (homolaterally). Imagine that your head is writing a figure 8 on the ceiling. Keep your spine straight but relaxed.

If you are applying too much weight, your mother hand will feel the receiver tense her hara—it will harden and tremble, even seem to push your hand away. In that case, lean back to lessen the pressure and wait for two or three seconds. If the hara relaxes and becomes loose, you can go deeper again by applying more weight first to the mother hand and then to the messenger hand. Always pay close attention to your mother hand—it will tell you how the receiver is reacting. You will eventually find the maximum body weight that the receiver can tolerate.

Never release the pressure entirely from one hand or the other. Pressure from just one hand can be unnecessarily painful and cause the hara to tighten immediately, which can also keep you from sensing the receiver's true condition.

Now, as the receiver exhales, lean in with the messenger hand once or twice in the area associated with the Heart meridian. When she exhales, move the messenger hand clockwise to the area associated with the Stomach meridian and lean in again. Continue in a clockwise direction until you reach the area of the Bladder meridian, about halfway around the hara, where you will switch mother and messenger hands for ease of movement. Then continue around the rest of the hara to the top of the solar plexus.

When you have finished, move your messenger hand around the hara again (switching at the area of the Bladder meridian), gradually decreasing the pressure from mother hand to messenger hand as you go. At the end, your hands will simply be resting on her hara, without applying any pressure at all.

MOTHER HAND AND MESSENGER HAND

When you touch a receiver, it is important always to use two hands and to increase or decrease pressure gradually from hand to hand. One hand (the mother hand) remains stationary, open and relaxed, sensitive to the receiver's reaction. The other hand (the messenger hand) moves along the pathways of energy, feeling where there is too much or too little, seeking to restore balance. The mother hand guides the messenger hand, directing its application of pressure, easing any discomfort the receiver might feel. The two hands work together to promote physical and spiritual balance in both the giver and the receiver.

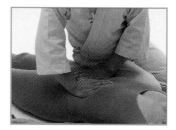
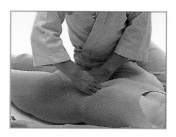

Fingers on the hara

For stronger penetration of the hara, you may use your fingers. First try four fingers, flat down. You may then sharpen them by applying only the tips. If you still need more penetration, go to three fingers. Using two fingers is the strongest technique of all. Don't use two fingers until you have practiced many times.

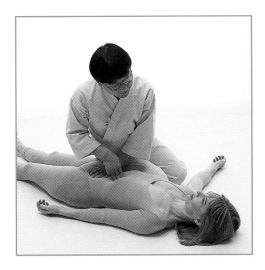

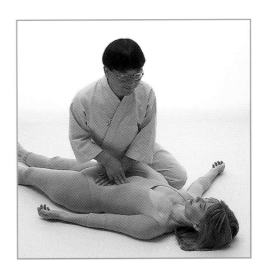

⊘ DON'T!

Here my body is too far away from the receiver. I will tire more easily and cannot adequately evaluate the meridian areas in the receiver's hara.

This is another mistake many people make. I am kneeling perpendicular to the receiver's hara, my back is rounded, and my neck and hands are tense. Approaching the receiver in this way produces homologous movement—going back and forth—which is abrupt and painful for the receiver. Because I am applying pressure with two hands simultaneously, she tightens her hara and I cannot evaluate it properly. (But my own body is so tense that I probably could not get a precise diagnosis anyway.)

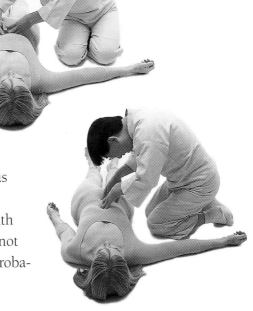

Returning to the hara

I return my hands to the hara after I've finished working on each part of the body. This gives me a chance to re-evaluate the receiver, to find out how effective the treatment is, and which areas still need attention.

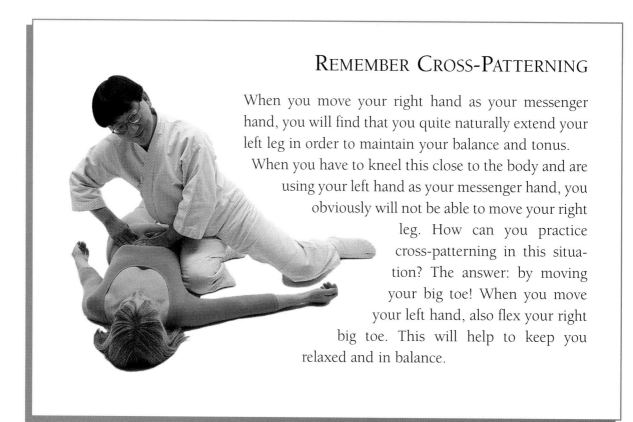

REMEMBER CROSS-PATTERNING

When you move your right hand as your messenger hand, you will find that you quite naturally extend your left leg in order to maintain your balance and tonus. When you have to kneel this close to the body and are using your left hand as your messenger hand, you obviously will not be able to move your right leg. How can you practice cross-patterning in this situation? The answer: by moving your big toe! When you move your left hand, also flex your right big toe. This will help to keep you relaxed and in balance.

UP AND DOWN THE LEGS

Sequence

- From the hara to the Stomach meridian in the upper legs

- Leg rotation

- Working the Spleen meridian

- Working the Gall Bladder meridian

    Elbow technique on the Gall Bladder meridian

- Working the Liver meridian

- Working the Stomach meridian, upper leg bent

    Elbow technique on the Stomach meridian

- Working the Kidney meridian

- Working the Stomach meridian, lower leg

- Foot rotation

- From one leg to the other

- Return from the legs to the hara

After my initial work on the hara, I move to the legs. Here, I follow a certain order of meridians, alternating between yang meridians (which travel from the top of the body down) and yin meridians (which travel from the bottom of the body up):

Stomach meridian, upper leg (yang)
Spleen meridian (yin)
Gall Bladder meridian (yang)
Liver meridian (yin)
Stomach meridian, upper leg bent (yang)
Kidney meridian (yin)
Stomach meridian, lower leg (yang)

You can find charts for locating these meridians in the booklet that accompanies this book.

Don't be too concerned at first about whether you are at exactly the right place on the meridian at every moment; it is enough to have a general idea of location and direction, and to focus instead on your movement.

You don't have to use every technique here (or even work along every meridian) in every session. As you gain experience, you will adapt your practice to the condition of the receiver. But you should try to learn as many of the techniques as you can, so that you can use them if you need them.

Remember, too, the principle of continuity. To provide a smooth transition, I rotate the leg after I finish one meridian and before starting on the next. The order of meridians, their alternation between yang and yin, and the rotation of the leg all contribute to beautiful and balanced movement. When you have mastered this sequence, you will find that your treatment looks like an elegantly choreographed dance.

From the hara to the Stomach meridian in the upper legs

The Stomach meridian is a yang meridian that runs down the front of the upper leg (see the meridian charts, page 2).

Move your right (messenger) hand from the hara to Stomach meridian tsubo #31 at the top of the receiver's right leg. As you move your right hand, be sure to also move your left (messenger) knee. Your mother hand remains on the left side of her hara above the navel.

Now, slowly raise your hips, turn your torso, and move both of your knees away from her body so that you are in the crawling position, perpendicular to her. Spread your knees apart so that you can move your left knee as you work down the leg.

Now, move your right (messenger) hand along the Stomach meridian down to the knee, around the area of tsubo #34 (see the meridian charts, page 2). Using either your palm or your thumb, lean into each of the major tsubos on the meridian for five to seven seconds. As your hand moves, so will your left (messenger) knee—you will be crawling sideways. Move your hara in a figure 8 pattern as you lean into the tsubos.

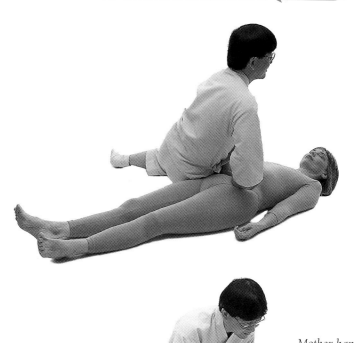

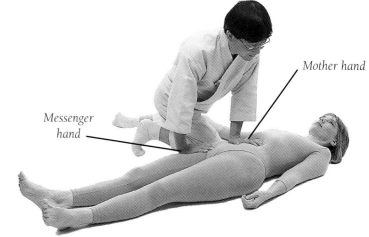

Mother hand

Messenger hand

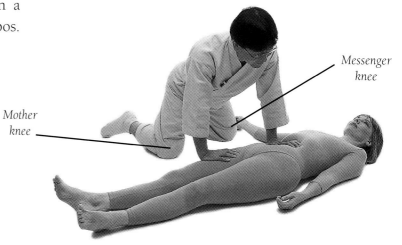

Messenger knee

Mother knee

DON'T!

This is a mistake some practitioners make when working on the legs. Because I am in a sitting—rather than a crawling—position, I cannot move from my hara and, therefore, end up pressing with my fingers and thumbs. When I bend my back and tense my muscles to try to increase the pressure, I cause pain to both myself and the receiver.

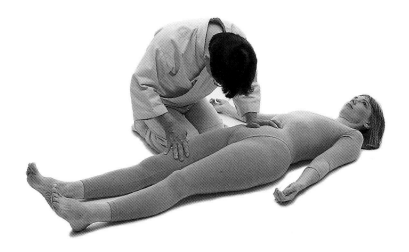

Occasionally, I see a practitioner raise one leg. This position disturbs the cross-patterning movement because the giver's body is twisted and the knee cannot be moved. When knee and hand movements cannot be coordinated, continuity is lost.

Leg rotation

After you finish working each meridian, you rotate the leg. Rotation gives you a number of advantages:

◆ It enables you to evaluate the receiver's condition, to decide which meridians need more attention.

◆ It allows both the giver and the receiver an opportunity to rest.

◆ It gives you time to choose the next technique and to move into the appropriate position.

◆ It contributes to the continuity of the Ohashiatsu session by providing a transition from one technique to the next.

◆ It is a form of therapy in itself, an exercise for the leg.

To rotate: Kneel diagonal to the receiver's torso. Keep your left hand (the mother hand) on her hara and, with your right hand and right knee pick up her right knee under the kneecap and bring it to *your* hara. Now, put your right knee down and bring your left knee up, with your foot flat on the floor. Holding her knee in place with your right hand, rotate her leg with your hara three to five times (see leg rotation directions on next page). Keep your hips raised and your spine straight. You may change the direction of the rotation if you feel resistance and tension in the leg; your mother hand will tell you how the receiver is reacting. If she is small and flexible and you want to stretch the leg more, you can move your left foot closer to her right arm and your right knee further up the side of her torso. Because you are using your entire body, it is easy to rotate, no matter how heavy the leg is.

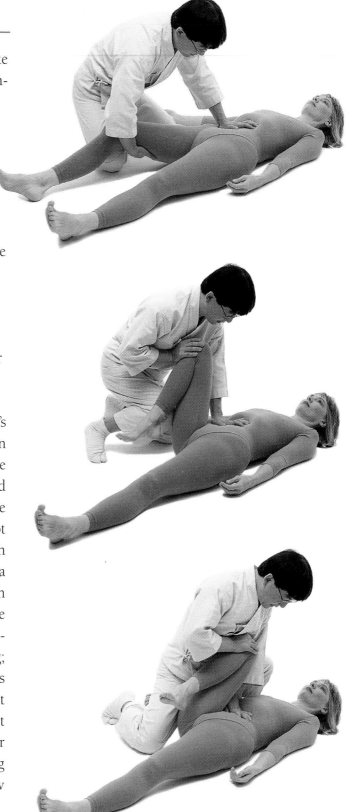

SINGLE LEG ROTATION

Leg rotation enables you to get a sense of the flexibility of the leg and the hip joint as you make the transition from one meridian to another. Although you may rotate the leg in either direction in small circles first, large rotations should be done with caution.

Because the hip needs time to respond, I recommend the rotation be done in stages. Bring the knee up toward the chest and lean in, stretching the leg as far as is comfortable for the receiver.

Then, release pressure slightly and continue the rotation until the knee is pointing to the shoulder closer to you and lean in again. Release and continue downward and around until the knee is pointing toward the opposite knee, and then lean in. Release pressure slightly, bring the knee up toward the opposite shoulder and lean in again. Listen with your mother hand on the hara, and ask the receiver if the rotation is too wide or the stretch too deep.

⊘ DON'T!

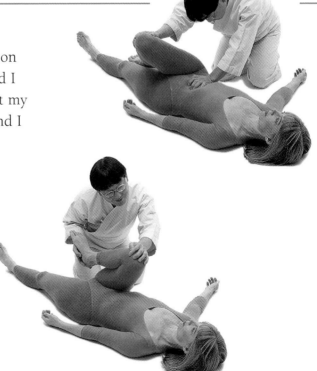

Here, I am sitting down with both knees on the floor instead of having one raised, and I am not holding the receiver's knee against my hara. In this position, my back is tense and I cannot achieve a wide enough rotation. I could damage my back and neck.

When I hold the leg with two hands (instead of keeping one hand on the hara) I cannot evaluate the receiver. Also, I lose cross-patterning movement.

Working the Spleen meridian

One of the principles of Ohashiatsu is to move your body before you move the receiver's body, to prepare yourself before you prepare the receiver. If you don't, you can waste time and energy in unnecessary movement. This principle is important to follow after each leg rotation, when you move to the next meridian.

After you have finished rotating the leg, lower it back to the floor, outstretched; move your body so that you are perpendicular to the receiver and put both knees on the floor. Now you are in position to work the Spleen meridian, a yin meridian that runs from the big toe up along the inside of the leg (see the meridian charts, page 3). Bring the receiver's right knee to rest on your right knee, the mother knee. (Your left hand, the mother hand,

stays on her hara but moves just below the navel.)

Since this is a yin meridian, travelling from the bottom of the body to the top, you begin work on it by putting your right palm on her right ankle, around Spleen #5. Your hand then moves up the inside of the leg along the shin bone to the top of her thigh, around Spleen #13. Use your palm three times along the meridian, then use your thumb three times.

Be sure that your left knee moves along with your hand. If the receiver is tall and heavy, you may be able to use your right elbow on the Spleen meridian in her upper leg, but do so with extreme care (see "Elbow Technique," pages 60–61), because it is a sensitive area. Never use the elbow on the lower leg.

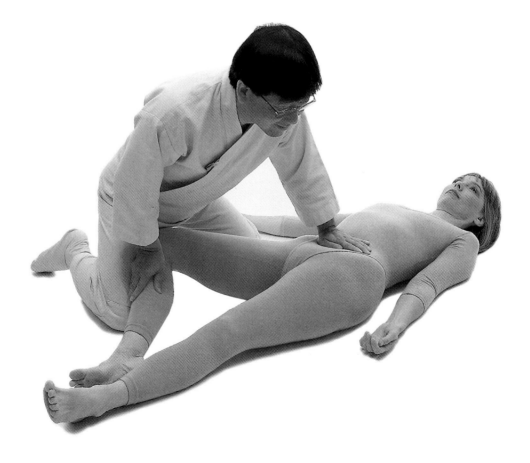

Working the Gall Bladder meridian

After you have finished working the Spleen meridian, raise your right knee and get into position to rotate the receiver's leg. After rotation, return to a kneeling position perpendicular to the receiver and bring her leg to rest on your right knee.

The Gall Bladder meridian is a yang meridian that runs down the outside of the leg to the fourth toe (see the meridian charts, page 6). Slide your mother hand (your left hand) to the upper left-hand corner of her hara.

Begin around Gall Bladder #29 or #30 at the top of the upper leg. Work down the meridian with your right palm three times, then with your thumb three times to the area of Gall Bladder #33 at the knee. At each of the major tsubos, raise your hips, lean toward the meridian (keeping your spine straight), and bring your hara toward her leg to increase the pressure.

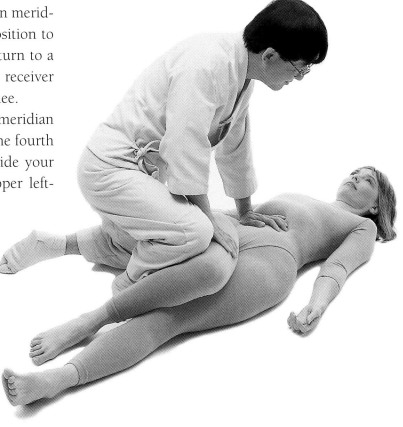

⊘ DON'T!

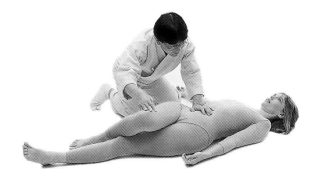

If I sit down, I can't lean from my hara, which makes it difficult to stretch the receiver's leg and to apply adequate pressure.

ELBOW TECHNIQUE

In Ohashiatsu, we usually use the hands—palms, fingers, or thumbs. But occasionally, when a receiver wants or needs deeper and stronger penetration, I use my forearms and elbows. When I use my elbows, I can keep my spine straight and relaxed and lean from my hara more easily than when I use my thumbs. So, using my elbows gives me a chance to rest even as it allows me to bring my body weight more fully to the receiver. It also gives variety to a session.

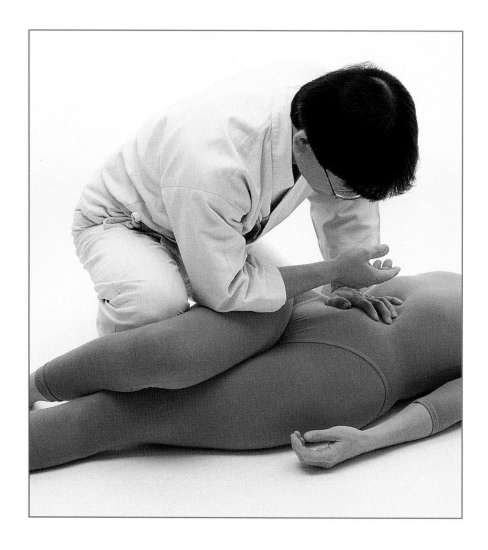

Elbow technique on the Gall Bladder meridian

Place your right elbow at the top of the receiver's upper leg, around Gall Bladder tsubo #30, keeping the forearm extended, palm up, with a relaxed hand. Bring your body gravity first to her hara and then, as she exhales, slowly shift to her leg . If your mother hand tells you that she can tolerate more, raise your hips and lean closer to her. Next, slowly bring your forearm toward your shoulder so that the pressure gradually becomes concentrated in your elbow. I call this *sharpening the elbow.*

Work down the meridian with your elbow to the knee, around Gall Bladder tsubo #33. Since elbow technique is so powerful, your movement should be slow and sensitive; always listen to the mother hand.

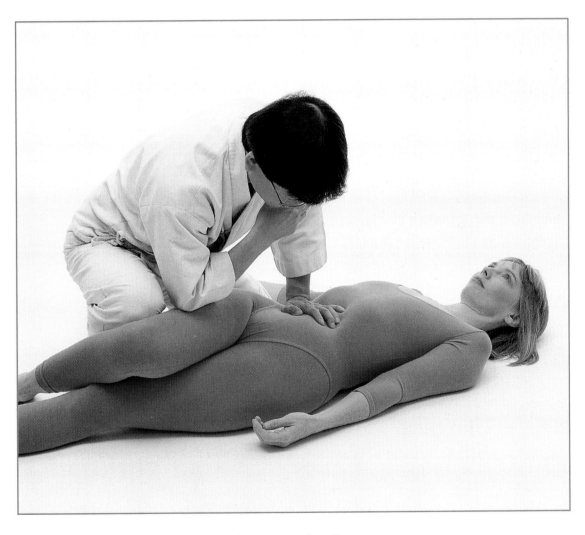

Sharpening the elbow

Working the Liver meridian

The Liver meridian is a yin meridian that runs from the big toe up the inside of the leg (see the meridian charts, page 6).

When you've finished the Gall Bladder meridian, rotate the receiver's leg and resume a kneeling position. As you bring the receiver's leg down, place her right foot against the inside of her left knee and support it on your right knee. Move your mother hand below the navel. Since this is another yin meridian, you will begin on the foot, around Liver tsubo #4. As you move your right hand up the meridian, if the receiver needs more of a stretch, you may move your right knee away from her body to stretch the leg. Using your palm or thumb, continue up to the knee around Liver tsubo #7 or #8.

When you want to go deeper on a tsubo, first lean toward the receiver, then lower your hips to stretch her leg more; hold for three to five seconds. Your mother hand will tell you how she is responding.

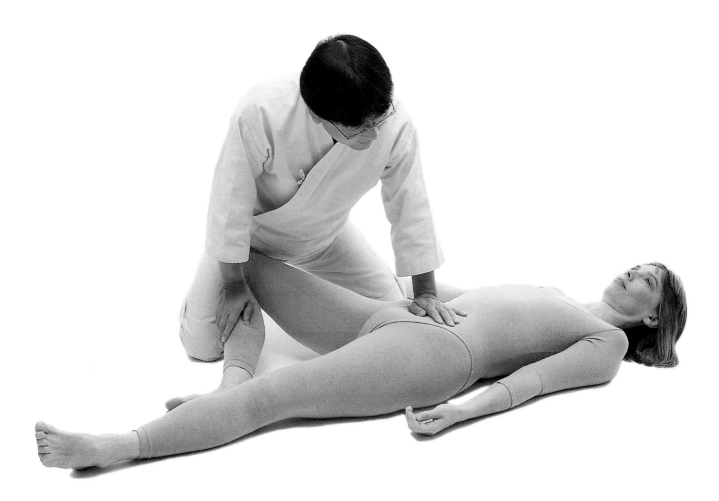

I have both hands on the meridian. Without a hand on the receiver's hara, I cannot tell if I'm causing her pain. And I cannot use cross-patterning; if I were to try to move my messenger knee, I would probably collapse.

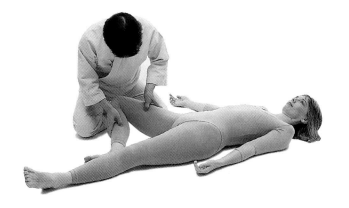

REPEATING TECHNIQUES— HOW OFTEN?

How often you work on a meridian— and whether you use your palm, thumb, or fingers—depends on how much surface area there is on a particular part of the body, how deeply you want to go, how much the receiver can tolerate, and how much time you have. I may say, "Do this two or three times," as a general guideline—but, in reality, you will decide.

INCREASING PRESSURE WITHOUT PRESSING

If you want to increase pressure on a tsubo, just lower your hips. When you do, you will naturally pull the receiver's leg toward your hara.

Also, always respect the purpose of the mother hand. Some tsubos—such as Spleen #6 and #10 on the leg—are very sensitive; if the receiver expresses discomfort, lean in more with the mother hand to counteract the feeling in the tsubo.

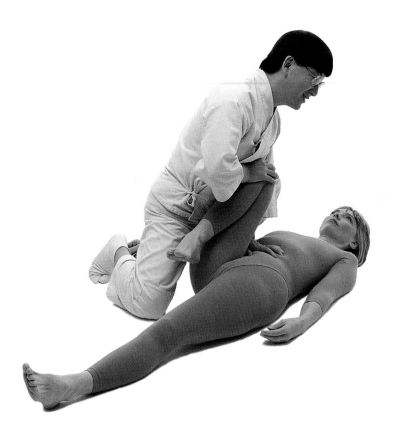

Working the Stomach meridian, upper leg bent

After you have finished the Liver meridian, pick up her leg and rotate it. As you finish rotating the leg, kneel down on your left knee, turn your torso perpendicular to the receiver, and bring your right knee around to catch the top of her foot. (Your hands will remain the same as for rotation.)

Lean toward her as you catch her foot, then bring your right knee toward your left knee so that her lower leg is bent under and the Stomach meridian is fully exposed. This position further stretches the Stomach meridian (see the meridian charts, page 2). In Ohashiatsu, we always try to stretch a meridian to the greatest possible extent to make sure energy can flow freely through it.

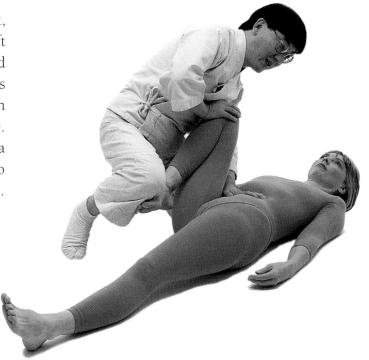

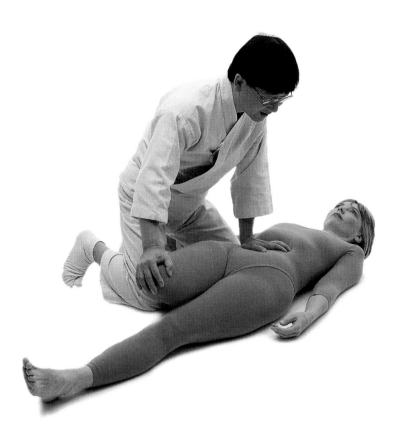

Support her right knee with your right leg. Slide your left hand (your mother hand) to the upper right corner of the hara, the area associated with the Stomach meridian. Next, palm down the upper leg of the Stomach meridian two or three times with your right hand to Stomach #34, just above the knee. Now, thumb down it two or three times. Keep a steady pressure with the mother hand and listen for the receiver's responses. You can stretch the leg further by leaning forward and sliding your right knee back slightly. Do this very slowly and carefully, always listening with your mother hand.

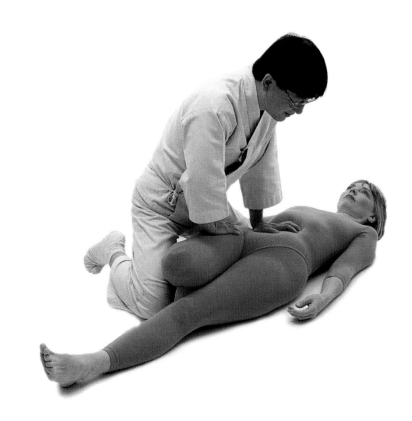

Elbow technique on the Stomach meridian

If the receiver's leg is long and heavy and stiff, you may want to use an elbow on the Stomach meridian.

Place your right elbow at the top of her leg, with your forearm relaxed and open at about a 90-degree angle. Moving from your hara, lean toward her leg by raising your hips. Now, slowly move your left knee back; as you do so, you will be applying more of your body weight. Slide your elbow from tsubo to tsubo. Repeat.

If you overstretch her leg, or apply too much pressure, she may tense her hara—a spasm you will feel in your mother hand. In that case, release the pressure and the stretch.

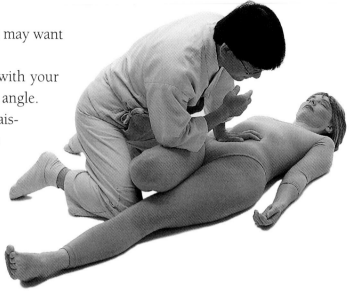

Working the Kidney meridian

After you rotate the receiver's leg, kneel a little further down her side in order to work on the Kidney meridian, a yin meridian that runs from the sole of the foot, up around the ankle, and up the inside of the leg (see the meridian charts, page 5).

Place your left (mother) hand on her hara just below the navel. Bend her leg and place her foot either on the floor or on her left knee, depending on which is most comfortable for her. In either case, support her right knee with your right leg.

Since the Kidney meridian is a yin meridian, you will be working from the foot up. Using the fingers of your right hand, begin on the sole of her foot between the bottom of the second and third toe, Kidney tsubo #1. Work up the entire leg along the meridian to the top of the thigh, around Kidney #12. When your mother hand tells you that she needs more stretch or pressure, lean toward her and move your right knee back.

Working the Stomach meridian, lower leg

As you finish rotating the receiver's leg and are lowering it to the floor, move your body down to be in position to work the Stomach meridian in her lower leg (see the meridian charts, page 2).

Because of the distance, you cannot reach the lower part of a fully extended leg while keeping your mother hand on her hara. So, for the Stomach meridian on the lower leg, I keep the thumb of my mother hand on the lower part of the kneecap, around Stomach tsubo #36, as I move the thumb of my messenger hand down the meridian to the ankle, near Stomach #41. When I move my thumb, I also move my messenger knee and lean from my hara. If you move in this way, you can bring your entire body weight to the Stomach meridian in the lower leg. The deeper you go, the more effective is your work.

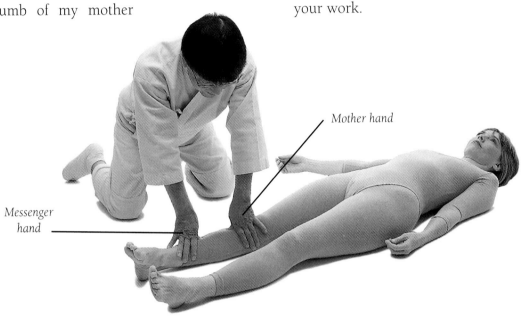

Mother hand

Messenger hand

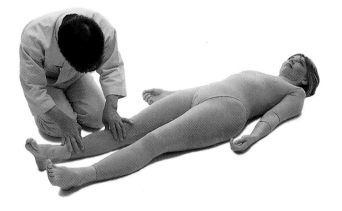

⊘ DON'T!

Don't kneel too close to the receiver's legs because you'll tend to lose your balance and not be able to use your entire body weight. Don't sit on your feet—you won't be able to move your messenger knee and will, therefore, disturb cross-patterning and lose continuity.

Foot rotation

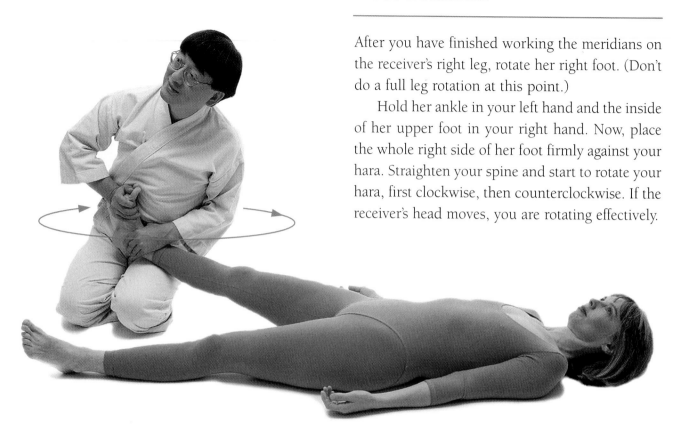

After you have finished working the meridians on the receiver's right leg, rotate her right foot. (Don't do a full leg rotation at this point.)

Hold her ankle in your left hand and the inside of her upper foot in your right hand. Now, place the whole right side of her foot firmly against your hara. Straighten your spine and start to rotate your hara, first clockwise, then counterclockwise. If the receiver's head moves, you are rotating effectively.

DON'T!

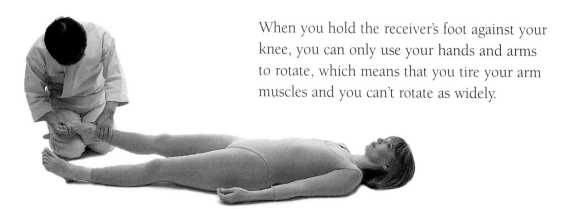

When you hold the receiver's foot against your knee, you can only use your hands and arms to rotate, which means that you tire your arm muscles and you can't rotate as widely.

From one leg to the other

This transition technique is especially good for the treatment of lower back pain.

As you finish rotating the receiver's foot, place it on the floor and move your body to face her feet. Grasp both ankles, straighten your arms, and lean back, pulling her legs toward you until her head moves a little bit. Repeat three times.

Now, bring her feet up against your hara and shift your hands to just below her kneecaps. When she exhales, raise your right knee and lean forward gradually, bending her knees toward her hara. Bend her legs toward her hara three times.

Next, with your hands still holding her knees, you will make the transition to her left side: Remove her feet from your hara, lean toward her, and place your right knee on the floor next to her left hip. Now, bring your left knee down beside your right knee. Keep your left hand on her knees, and move your right hand to her hara. With your left hand, extend her legs and lower them to the floor; don't let them drop.

Now, you are ready to work the Stomach meridian on her left upper leg, using your left hand as the messenger hand. Repeat all of the techniques in this section on the left leg, switching hands and knees—that is, when text calls for "right hand" or "right knee," you will be using your left ones.

Return from the legs to the hara

After you have finished working on the receiver's left leg and rotating the left foot, pick up both legs by the ankles and hold her feet against your hara. Bend her legs toward her hara and rotate them. As you do so, move around to her right side; hook your left arm under her legs and slowly lower her legs to the floor. Assume a seiza position, about midway up and parallel to the receiver's side, with both of your hands on her hara. Now you are ready to begin working on the arms.

OUT AND AROUND THE ARMS

Sequence

- From the hara to the arms

- Working the Heart Constrictor meridian

- From the Heart Constrictor meridian to the Heart meridian

- Working the Heart meridian

- From the Heart meridian to the Lung meridian

- Working the Lung meridian

- From one arm to the other

- From the Lung meridian to the Heart meridian

- From the Heart meridian to the Heart Constrictor meridian

- From the arms to the neck

In order to keep my own movements to a minimum when I am working on the arms, I reverse the order in which I work the meridians from one arm to the other. If I were to do them both in the same order, I would have to travel all the way to the other side of the receiver; by reversing the order, I can make a more efficient transition, just moving from shoulder to shoulder.

You will also notice that when I am working from behind the receiver's head, I cannot always keep one hand on the hara.

From the hara to the arms

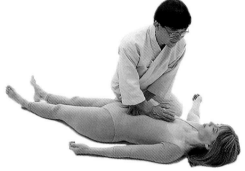

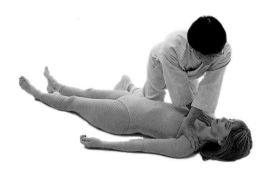

After you have finished evaluating the hara, slowly slide the side of your right hand up along the Conception Vessel meridian, in the center of the chest, and over toward the receiver's right shoulder. (Following the meridian allows you to tell where the receiver may have pain or discomfort in the torso.)

Grasp her shoulder with your thumb in the center of her armpit and your fingers over the top of her shoulder. Squeeze the shoulder slowly as you raise your hips and slide your left hand up the Conception Vessel meridian, over your right hand to her left shoulder, which you grasp in the same way as you did her right shoulder. Your arms are now crossed.

Lean toward her and move your hara in a figure 8 to loosen any tension in the shoulders. As you lean, move your knees further down beside her body so that when you begin working on her arm, you will have enough room to lean deeply from your hara.

⊘ DON'T!

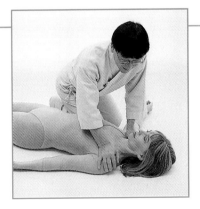

In my years of experience, I've discovered that small errors in technique can make a big difference.

Notice that I haven't crossed my arms. In order to begin the next technique, I will now have to move both hands, instead of only one; I will have lost continuity.

I've also failed to put my thumbs in her armpits; without a secure hold on her shoulders, I could easily slip off and fall on her as I bring my body weight forward. (I've had this embarrassing experience!)

In addition, my knees are too close to her arm; I can't lean far enough from my hara, and I end up having to bend my back and use my shoulders and arms, causing discomfort for both the receiver and me.

Working the Heart Constrictor meridian

The Heart Constrictor meridian is a yin meridian that runs from the armpit up the middle of the inner arm to the middle finger (see the meridian charts, page 5).

Hold the receiver's right shoulder with the thumb of your right hand (the mother hand) in the upper edge of the armpit, around the area of Heart Constrictor tsubo #2. Place your left hand (the messenger hand) on her upper arm beside your right hand. As you do this, get your body into the crawling position, making sure that your knees are far enough back to allow you to lean as deeply as possible.

Work along the meridian with your left palm or thumb two or three times, ending at Heart Constrictor #9, at the tip of the middle finger. Be sure that your right knee (the messenger knee) moves along with your left hand; your mother hand remains on the armpit.

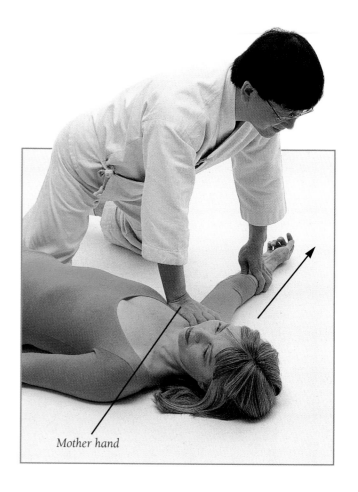

Mother hand

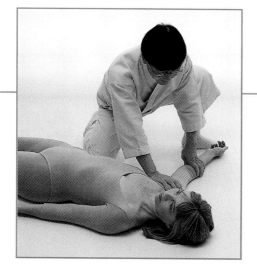

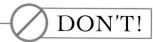

DON'T!

Here I've raised my mother knee. In this position I can't move my messenger knee easily as I work the meridian.

From the Heart Constrictor meridian to the Heart meridian

After I have finished working a meridian and before I go on to the next, I move the receiver's arm, to preserve continuity as I reposition myself.

After you finish working the Heart Constrictor meridian, keep your mother hand in place, and pick up the receiver's arm by the wrist with your left hand. From the kneeling position, raise your left knee and move your foot to be parallel to her body. In one movement lower your knee, stretch her arm up above her head, and bring it down to rest on your knee. With her arm in this position the Heart meridian is fully exposed and waiting for you.

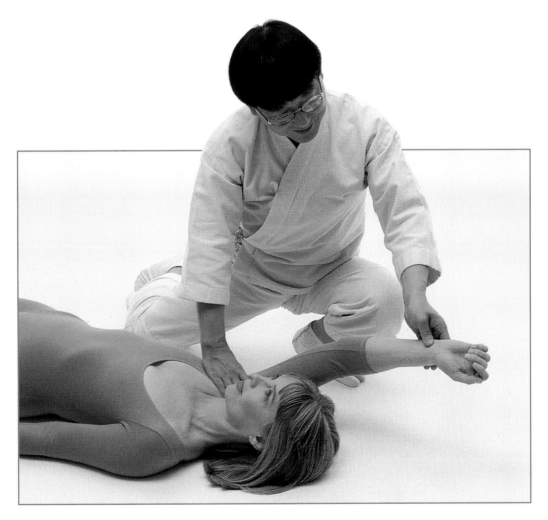

Repositioning the arm

Working the Heart meridian

The Heart meridian is a yin meridian that runs from the armpit along the innermost edge of the arm to the inside of the little finger, just below the nail (see the meridian charts, page 3).

The thumb of your right (mother) hand holds Heart meridian tsubo #1, at the base of the receiver's armpit while the fingers squeeze the armpit firmly. Be sure that your left knee supports her right elbow. (The elbow of some people who have a heart problem sits higher than normal and cannot lie flat on the floor when the arm is extended.)

Your left (messenger) hand will move up the meridian to her little finger at Heart # 9. Lean from your hara into each of the major tsubos along the way, to stretch the arm. When you come to the elbow, stretch it carefully against your knee.

Be sure your right knee moves sideways when your left hand moves. Moving your messenger knee—one of the forms of cross-patterning in

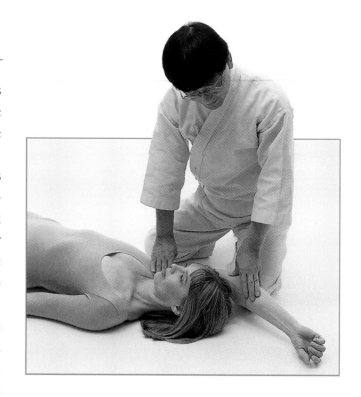

Ohashiatsu—will help you maintain balance and reduce fatigue.

Work the meridian a few times with either your palm or your thumb.

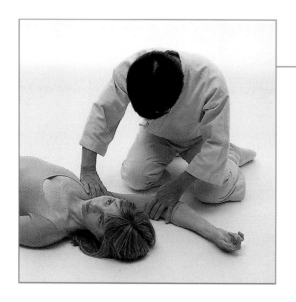

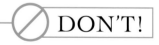
DON'T!

Because I'm neither holding Heart tsubo #1 firmly nor supporting the elbow, I can't stretch her arm along the meridian as fully as I should. And because I'm sitting too far away, my back is rounded.

From the Heart meridian to the Lung meridian

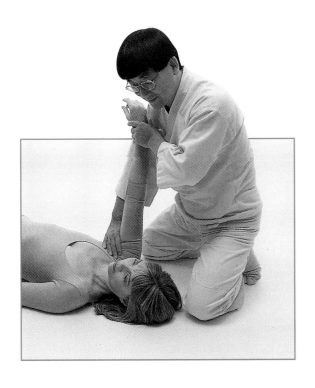

After you have worked along the Heart meridian, you will be repositioning the arm—and yourself—for work on the Lung meridian.

Pick up the receiver's right arm at the wrist with your left (messenger) hand; keep your right (mother) hand in place, holding her right armpit. Next, bring her right arm to rest on your right shoulder and, as you do so, move on your knees into position behind her right shoulder, about a torso-length back.

Now, switch hands (see lower left photograph), so that your right hand slides up to hold her wrist and your left hand (now becoming the mother hand) slides down over her collarbone. Now, lower her arm to the floor, palm up and perpendicular to her body.

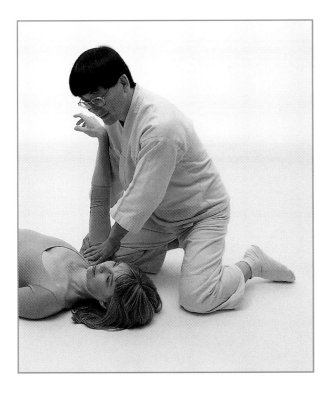

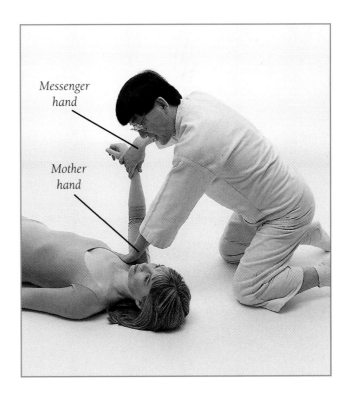

Messenger hand

Mother hand

Working the Lung meridian

The Lung meridian is a yin meridian that runs along the inside of the arm from the collar bone to the tip of the thumb, just below the nail (see the meridian charts, page 2).

You should now be in a crawling position, with your knees spread and your toes relaxed. Your left (mother) hand holds Lung tsubo #1, about an inch below the outer end of the receiver's collarbone. Your right (messenger) hand moves next to your left one, at the top of the arm. Bring your weight to your left hand and slowly shift to your right hand in a figure 8 pattern until the weight is evenly distributed, to minimize any discomfort the receiver might feel. Stay for two or three seconds. Begin working along the meridian with your right hand, using either your palm or your thumb, up to Lung #11 on the thumb. Repeat two or three times. Use a small figure 8 movement as you lean into each tsubo and remember to move your left knee as your right hand moves up the meridian.

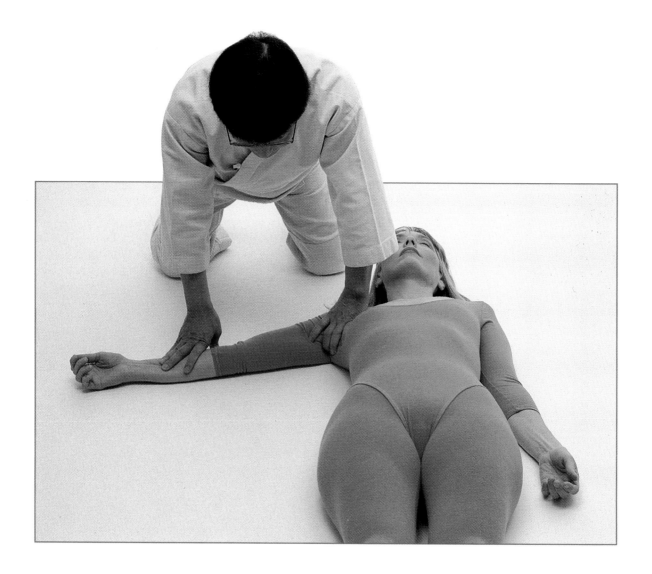

From one arm to the other

After you have finished the Lung meridian on the right arm, you will next get into position to work on the left arm.

Release your right hand from her thumb, cross your right arm over your left arm, and put your right palm just below the receiver's left collarbone at Lung #1. As you cross your hands, move sideways on your knees so that you are centered between her shoulders.

Next, squeeze her armpits and lean forward toward her shoulders, moving your hara in a figure 8. When you do this, you will be able to tell if the receiver has remaining stiffness or tension in either of her shoulders.

Now, release your left hand (which becomes the messenger hand) and bring it beside your right one as you move sideways and resume a crawling position, to begin work on the Lung meridian of the left arm. Proceed in the same manner as described on the previous page.

When you make this transition, always remember to cross your arms and hold the receiver's armpits. Otherwise you'll have to move your hands twice and be in danger of losing contact with her.

You work the Lung, Heart, and Heart Constrictor meridians on the left arm in much the same way you worked those on the right arm—but in the reverse order and from slightly different positions. In order to minimize your movements, you will work the Lung meridian while facing the receiver's feet. You will return to that position when you work on the Heart Constrictor meridian so that you can make an easier transition to working on the neck.

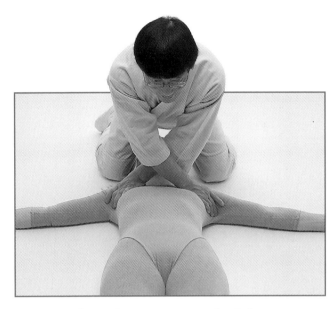

Making the transition to the left arm

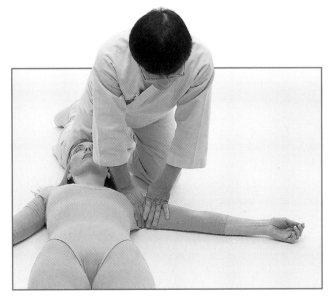

Starting work on the Lung meridian

From the Lung meridian to the Heart meridian

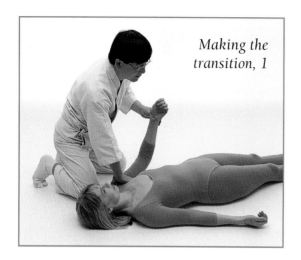

Making the transition, 1

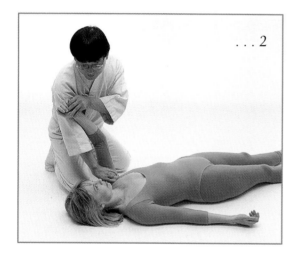

. . . 2

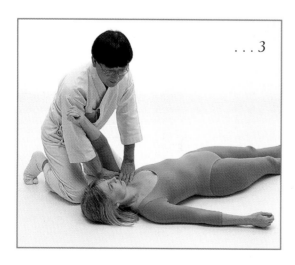

. . . 3

After you have finished the Lung meridian, pick up the receiver's left arm by the wrist with your left (messenger) hand and put it on your right shoulder.

Squeeze her armpit at Heart #1 with your right (mother) hand, which has remained in place on top of her shoulder. Make sure her arm is resting securely against you, then release your left hand and move it down to grasp her armpit. Intertwine the fingers of both hands and squeeze her shoulder.

Now, move into a kneeling position perpendicular to her shoulder as you slide your right hand up to her wrist and lower her arm. Rest her elbow on your right knee. Your right hand is now the messenger hand, and your left hand is the mother hand (at Heart tsubo #1). You are ready to work the Heart meridian on the left arm. Follow the directions on page 74, substituting "right" for "left" as you read the text.

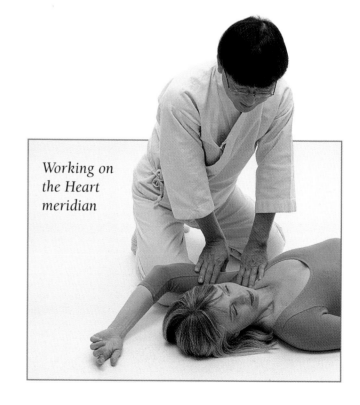

Working on the Heart meridian

From the Heart meridian to the Heart Constrictor meridian

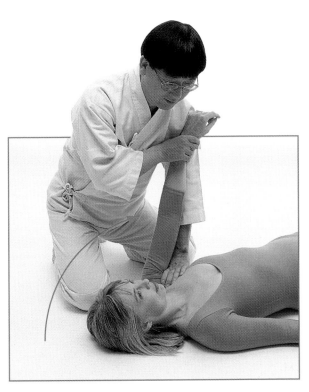

Making the transition

After you have finished the Heart meridian, you will resume the position you were in for the Lung meridian.

Pick up the receiver's left arm by the wrist with your right hand and bring it to your left shoulder. With her arm resting on your shoulder, bring your right (messenger) hand down beside your left (mother) hand and squeeze.

Now, with your left hand, lower her arm, palm up and perpendicular to her body—as you move yourself around so that you are in a crawling position, parallel to her and facing her feet. Be sure your knees are far enough from her arm so that you can lean deeply.

Your left hand is now the messenger hand, and your right hand is the mother hand. You are now in position to work the Heart Constrictor meridian (see p. 72).

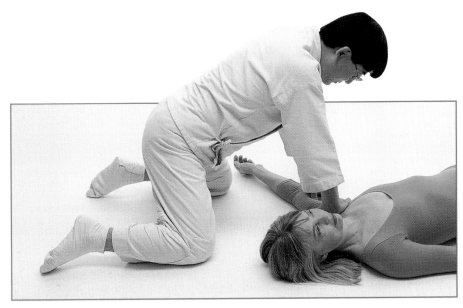

Working on the Heart Constrictor meridian

From the arms to the neck

When you have finished the Heart Constrictor meridian, keep your right (mother) hand in place and cross over it with your left hand, which you use to grasp her right collarbone. As you are crossing your hands, move your knees until you are directly behind her head. Lean toward her shoulders and move your hara in a figure 8. This will help you evaluate the receiver's condition before you go on to work on the neck.

You will notice that this is the same movement you used (from the opposite side, of course) in making the transition from one arm to the other (see "From one arm to the other," page 77). In Ohashiatsu, the familiarity and ease of transitions are comforting to the receiver and enhances a sense of trust.

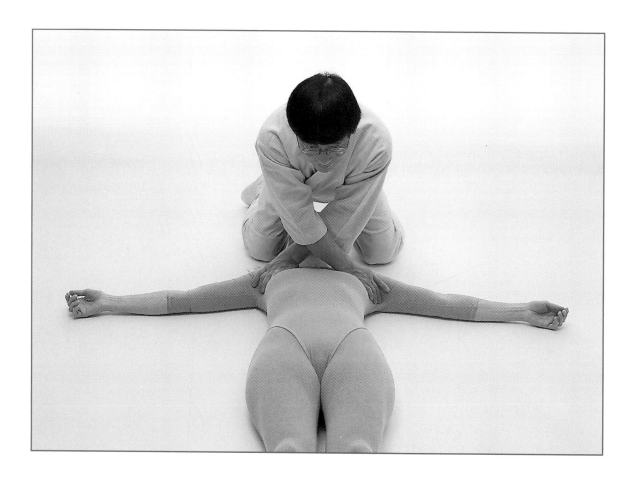

HANDS ON THE NECK

The neck is one of the most sensitive and difficult areas to work on. Many meridians and nerves run through it, as well as important arteries and veins, the larynx, and respiratory and digestive tubes. This narrow "bottleneck" area—caught between a heavy cranium, representing intellect and spirituality, and the torso, representing health and vitality—is a crucial part of our bodies. It is not surprising that many people hold tension and stress in the neck.

Treating the neck requires a sensitive touch, knowledge of the neck's anatomy, and highly developed technique. A Japanese proverb says it takes three years to master techniques for the back and hips, but eight years to master techniques for the neck. The way you treat the neck immediately reveals your experience and sensitivity, and how much the receiver trusts you. Unless the receiver is totally relaxed, you cannot give deep, effective Ohashiatsu to the neck. Trying to force treatment can be dangerous. Mutual trust, respect, and sensitivity are essential on both sides.

In this section, I offer all the techniques I have developed for the neck during my years of practice. You will never use all of them in a single session; using three to five techniques each time should be sufficient. Try to provide balance and variety in your choice: Alternate center stretches with side stretches, for instance. If you find that the receiver resists a certain technique, try a gentler one, one that does not stretch as much or penetrate as deeply.

Ideally, you should learn every one of these techniques, so that you will have as much choice as possible. The more techniques you are acquainted with, the more efficient you will be. Make sure you are completely relaxed; if you feel hurried or tense, you should work on a less sensitive part of the body. Ohashiatsu to the neck is a test of how relaxed, calm, and centered you are as a giver. The receiver will let you know.

Preparation: Palms over eyes

After you have made the transition from the arms to the neck, you will be kneeling directly behind the receiver's head with your arms crossed and on her shoulders. Release your hands. Make sure they are clean and dry. If you need to, rub down your palms several times to energize and warm them; then put them over the receiver's eyes.

Close your eyes briefly to calm your mind, and synchronize your breathing with that of the receiver's. When her eyelashes stop moving, she is ready to receive. You will repeat this gesture as a transition from technique to technique while working on the neck.

If her face and neck feel warm, she could be reacting to your cold hands. Rub them down again—or use a thin cotton scarf to cover her face and neck (see "Using a scarf," pages 94–95). You can also use a scarf when your hands are oily or sweaty. Ideally, you want your hands to be warmer and drier than the receiver's face.

You will use the squatting position (see Chapter 2) more often when you work on the neck because it allows you to move your entire body in a small area. You will usually keep one leg raised, to give you greater flexibility as you stretch. Always keep your spine straight and move from your hara; don't use your arm and finger muscles. Remember cross-patterning.

You will also find that there is sometimes less distinction here between mother and messenger hand—because the area is so small, and for many of the stretches both hands remain stationary.

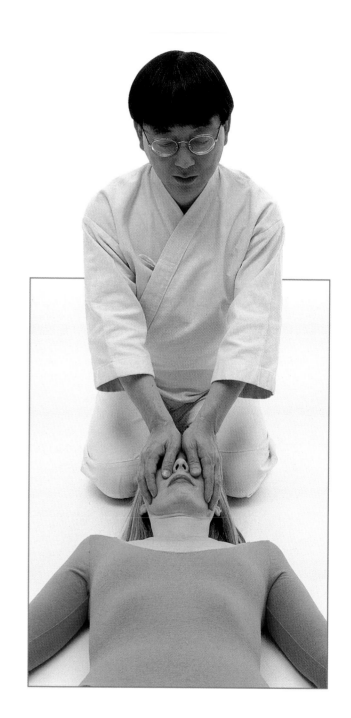

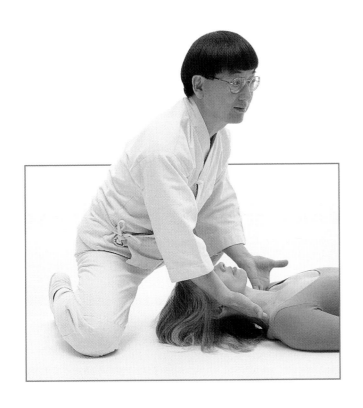

Evaluating with a two-handed center stretch

You should use this technique as you begin work on the neck, to evaluate the receiver's condition. It will tell you which side of the neck is tense and whether she has arthritis or any abnormality of the vertebrae. If an abnormality exists, don't continue. Gently bring the neck session to an end and move on to another part of the body.

After your palms have been resting on her eyes for a few seconds, slowly slide them back over her temples, behind her ears, and down to her shoulders, around Gall Bladder tsubo #21 (see the meridian charts, page 6). Keep one leg raised (if you are right-handed, it is natural to raise your left leg) and your spine and arms straight. Next, slowly slide both hands up her neck to the bottom of her cranium, where you feel a dip. Now, slide your hands back down to her shoulders; move your hara as you move your hands. When your fingers are sliding up the neck, pull the neck toward you—pull until you can see her big toes move. Repeat several times. (But if the receiver tenses, release immediately.)

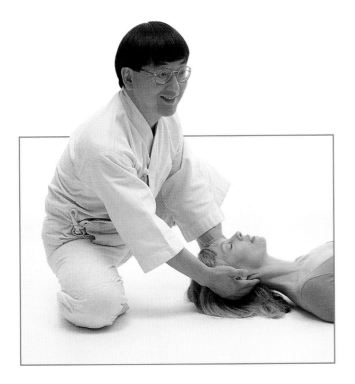

⊘ DON'T!

Here I haven't kept one leg raised. The kneeling position forces me to use muscle power to stretch the receiver's neck. You can see the tension in my rounded spine. Also, it isn't pleasant for the receiver to have me breathing directly into her face.

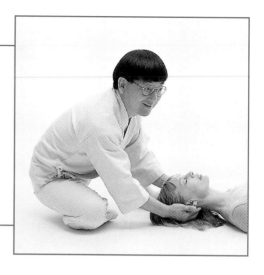

Loosening up the neck with a figure 8 movement

This is an easy and safe technique for loosening up the neck.

Apply both hands to the bottom of her cranium and lift her head slightly. Raise one leg; keep your spine and arms straight. Next, move your hips in a figure 8 pattern and as you do so, her head will also naturally move in a figure 8 pattern (again, imagine that you are drawing a figure 8 on

the ceiling with your head). If she resists, change direction. (Don't tell her to relax—in my experience, the receiver tenses up more when told to relax.) While she is breathing out, pull her body toward you. Repeat several times, then slide your hands up over her forehead, and place your palms over her eyes once again.

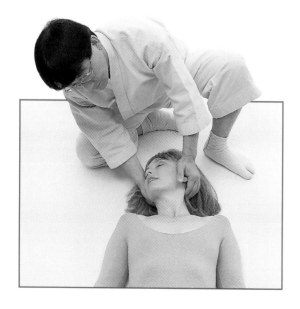

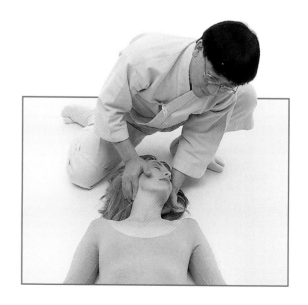

SIDE STRETCHES

Using two hands

This is a good technique for problems in the neck and lower backache.

    With your left leg raised, put your right hand (fingers flat) on the receiver's left shoulder, so that her head is resting on your forearm. Place your left palm on the back of her head to support it. Synchronize your breathing with hers. As she exhales, slowly raise your hara and lean toward her left side, in order to stretch her neck in that direction. Repeat a few times, releasing at the end of each stretch. If her neck is flexible, you can bring your right knee closer to her, to stretch more fully.

    Switch hand and leg positions and repeat this technique on the other side of the neck.

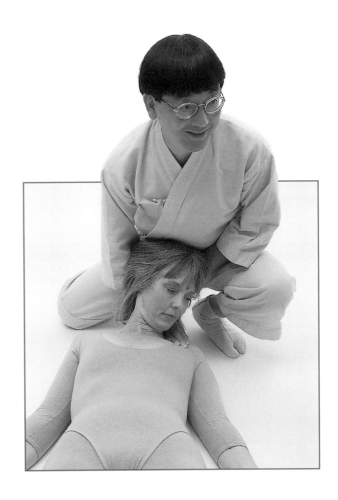

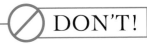

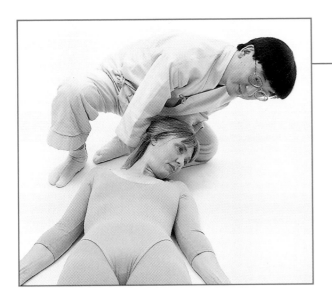

Here, I have the wrong leg raised, which makes me lean too far to one side and become unstable. If you feel insecure in your position, you will tense up and the receiver's neck may tighten in response. And again, because my back is rounded, not straight, I am straining my spine and possibly doing damage to my body.

Using the side of the hand

In this technique you apply the side of your hand (the index finger side) in between the vertebrae on the side of the neck.

Raise your left leg. Hold the right side of the receiver's head with your right palm. Keep the fingers of your left hand straight and together, and place the index finger side of your hand across the back left *side* of her neck. Start at the bottom of her cranium; you can rest your thumb on her jaw for support.

When she breathes out, use your right hand and your hara to bring her head toward your left hand. In order to stretch further, raise your left heel to press your knee against your elbow. Now,

bring her head back to the center, slide your index finger down her neck in between the next two vertebrae, and then bring her head back to your index finger again. Repeat at five places along the neck, and do the whole sequence three to five times. (But if there is any resistance in the neck, don't continue.) Keep her face up and her head parallel to the floor. Always be sure to use your hara movement to move her head.

You can also practice this technique with your thumb, knuckle, or the tips of your fingers, for variety.

Switch hand and leg positions, and repeat on the other side.

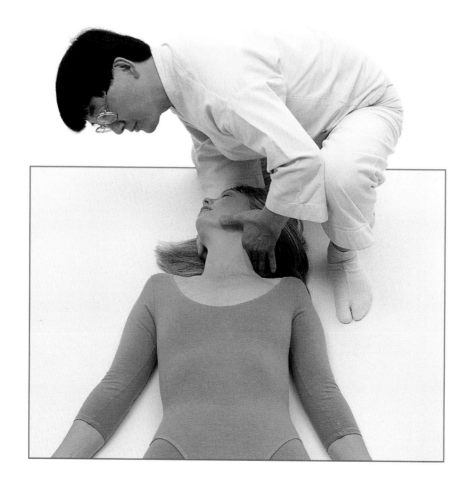

PALMS OVER EYES

Don't ever rush an Ohashiatsu neck routine. Each time you finish one technique, return your palms to the receiver's eyes and rest them there for about 10 seconds. Both of you will feel more relaxed.

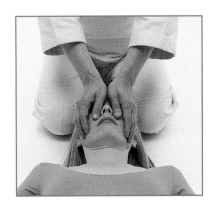

CENTER STRETCHES

With one hand squeezing

This technique is good for headache, lower backache, and insomnia.

The Bladder meridian runs from the inner corner of the eye up the forehead, then down the back of the head and neck (see the meridian charts, page 4).

Hold up the upper part of the receiver's head with the palm of your left (mother) hand around the area of Bladder #10 (see the meridian charts). With your right leg raised, squeeze the back of her neck with your right hand along the Bladder meridian, on both sides of the cervical vertebrae (see the meridian charts, page 4). As you squeeze, lift her head with your left hand and raise your hips and torso, in order to stretch her neck. Move your hand down the neck in this manner, squeezing the Bladder meridian and stretching. If at any point the receiver cannot tolerate the amount of stretching, immediately lower her head to relax her.

Note that the receiver must completely relax her neck and back—her entire body—for this technique to be effective. Check her fingers and toes. If they are open, she has surrendered to your touch. If they are curled up, she still has some tension; don't continue.

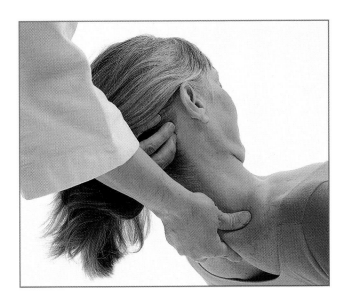

Using both arms

Cross your arms and place your palms on the receiver's shoulders. Rest her head on your arms and raise one leg. When she exhales, slowly raise your hips and her head. Don't try to raise her head with your arms only; use your entire body. At the furthest limit of the stretch, push her shoulders down with your fingers and lean toward her again. (But don't breathe directly on her.) Repeat.

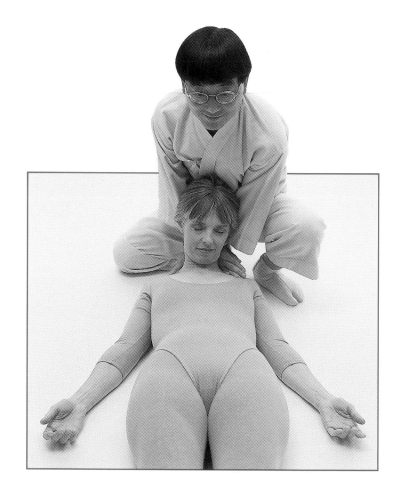

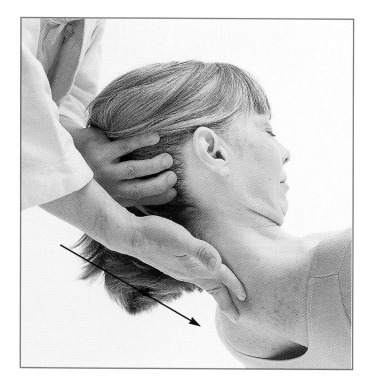

With one hand sliding

This feels much different from using both arms—it stretches the neck more and gives deeper pressure.

Put your left hand on the back of the receiver's head, and hold it up. Raise your right leg. Place your right fingers at the bottom of her cranium, around Bladder tsubo #10. When she exhales, slowly slide your fingers down to the base of her neck and raise your hips and torso.

Repeat slowly several times (always when she exhales).

With one hand on shoulder

This is even more powerful than the previous technique.

Put your left palm on the receiver's left shoulder and your right hand at the bottom of her cranium. Raise your left leg. When she exhales, raise your hips to raise her head, and slide your right hand down to the base of her neck. You may squeeze with your hand to increase the pressure, and lean toward her shoulder to increase the stretch.

Repeat a couple of times; then switch your hand and leg positions and repeat again.

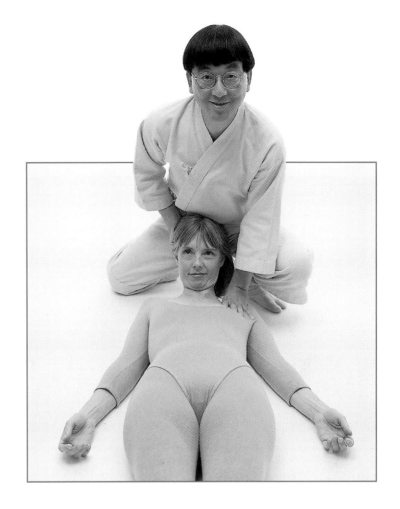

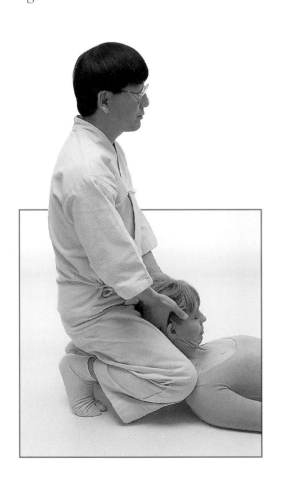

With knees on shoulders

This is the most powerful stretching technique for the neck. Use it when both you and the receiver are very flexible.

Get into a squatting position and bring your knees to the receiver's shoulders. Make sure your weight is on your toes and not on your knees. Keep your spine straight. Hold her head with both hands behind her ears, fingers pointing downward. Now, raise your hips toward the ceiling and stretch her neck. Note that the receiver's head does not touch your body.

If you find that using both knees together is too difficult for you, you can use one knee at a time (and keep the other knee on the floor).

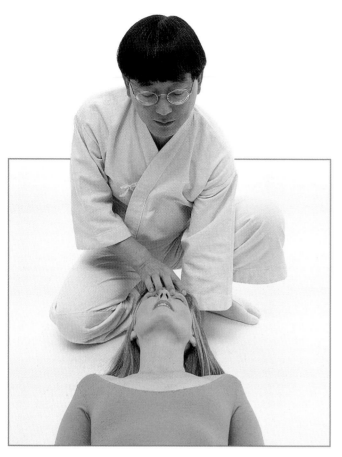

Front view

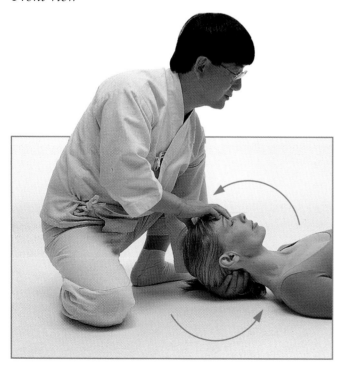

Side view

"Vacuum" stretch

When I do this technique on someone, I jokingly tell her that I am vacuuming her brains into mine, which will make her feel lighter and me feel smarter.

Be sure her eyes are closed. Raise one leg. Put the tip of your right index finger and right middle finger on the inner corners of the eye sockets on both sides of her nose, around Bladder meridian #1 (see the meridian charts, page 4). Pull slightly upward, toward the eyebrows.

Meanwhile, place the four fingers of your left hand, palm up, on the back of her head, with the tips of your third and fourth fingers on Bladder #10 tsubos, just below the second cervical vertebra, and the tip of your little and index fingers on Gall Bladder #20 tsubos at the base of the skull, just behind the ear. Support the full weight of her head on your fingers.

Now, pull your right fingers toward you and push your left fingers slightly toward her shoulder; don't actually move your fingers—just redirect their pressure. This will cause her jaw to relax and open slightly. Hold for a couple of minutes while you meditate together. (You can gently vibrate her head in this position by vibrating your fingers. Sometimes I add a vibrating sound in a low voice.)

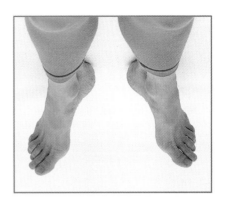

WATCH THE RECEIVER'S BIG TOE
Whenever you're giving Ohashiatsu to the neck, observe whether the receiver's feet are moving. The relationship between the feet should look more balanced as the hip sockets open. Pay special attention to the big toe opposite the side you are working on—when it moves, you know your technique is influencing the entire body.

"Sinking-head" stretch

This is an effective technique for especially tense and nervous people.

Kneel down with your knees together or apart, whichever is most comfortable for you. With your hands on the floor, palms up and fingers raised, rest the bottom of the receiver's cranium on your finger tips. Hold for a couple of minutes. Feel the pulse in her cranium; notice whether she is relaxing her neck. As her head sinks onto your fingers,

her pulse will become more regular, steady, and deep. Tell her to keep her mouth open and her eyes closed.

If you shift your wrists slightly toward her shoulders, her jaw will open even more. Hold for another couple of minutes.

Sometimes, I slowly wave my fingers to vibrate the head and intensify the sensation.

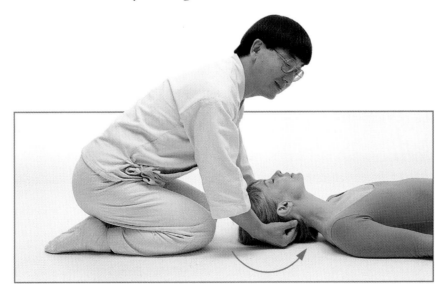

SIDE-TO-SIDE STRETCHES

Turning the face

Place the fingers of both hands behind the receiver's ears, with your thumbs resting on her cheekbones. Keep your arms relaxed and straight; raise one knee. When she's breathing out, turn her face to the side opposite your raised knee. Repeat several times, always when she exhales.

If you feel resistance in her neck, turn her face back up and wait for two or three seconds, then try again; don't force the stretch. Be sure you are not just turning with your hands; move your body in the direction of the turn, and her head will naturally turn, too. Don't move her head abruptly or try to crack her neck vertebrae—that can be extremely dangerous. Stay in tonus; the more relaxed you and the receiver are, the more you will be able to stretch.

Now, turn her face to the other side, lower your raised leg, and raise the other one. Repeat the technique a few times in this direction.

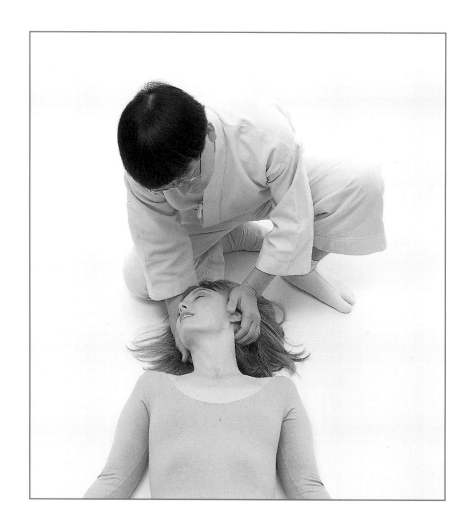

Face-up stretch

Position yourself so that you are slightly diagonal to the receiver's head.

First, roll her head slowly from side to side and note any resistance. If one side seems looser than the other, begin on that side.

If you are beginning on the right side, raise your left leg and place your right palm on the right side of her head; then cross your left arm over your right arm and put your left hand on her right shoulder. Keep her face up. When she exhales, lean toward her and move her head toward her left shoulder while you stretch her right shoulder with your left palm. Repeat three to five times. When you have stretched as far as you can, release the shoulder a little bit and then stretch farther. If you are not sure how much is comfortable for the receiver, ask her.

Now, switch hand and leg positions and stretch the other side.

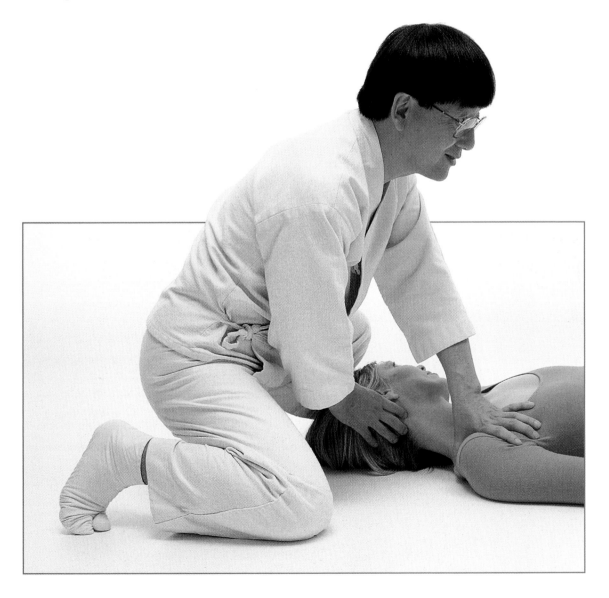

USING A SCARF

If a receiver is especially flexible and can tolerate more stretching, I sometimes use a scarf, a technique I developed to help me stretch more evenly and comfortably. Some receivers like the feeling of the fabric. I use a thin, cotton, rectangular Japanese scarf, about an arm's length long and about a foot wide.

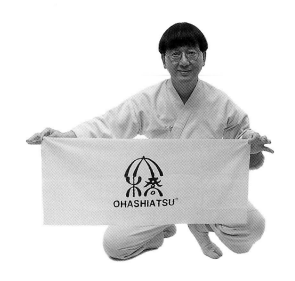

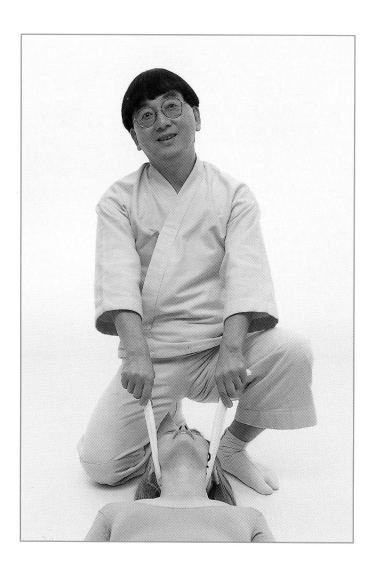

Center stretch

Slip the scarf under the receiver's head and down to the base of her neck; hold both ends and keep your arms straight and relaxed. Raise either leg. When she is breathing out, raise your hips and slowly slide the scarf up her neck to the bottom of her cranium; be sure that your arms remain straight.

Return the scarf to the base of her neck and repeat this technique several times, as she exhales, until you notice that her big toes move. That indicates that the stretch has affected her entire body; you've done a good job.

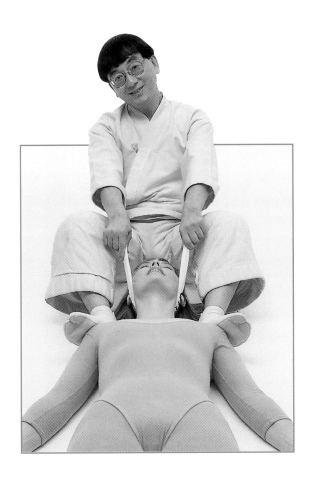

"Bicycle" stretch

I call this the "bicycle" technique. It's more powerful than the center stretch.

Sit back from the receiver's head and put one
foot on each of her shoulders. Hold the scarf
around the bottom of her cranium. Keeping your
arms straight, pull her neck toward you. When
she exhales, press one of her shoulders with your
foot; when she inhales, release. When she exhales
again, press the other shoulder; when she inhales
again, release. Continue, alternating shoulders.
Your feet and legs will be moving as though you
are riding a bicycle. Keep her head centered
between your legs and keep her face up. Watch
her big toes to be sure the technique is working:
When you press her left shoulder, her left big toe
should move, and vice versa.

Side stretch

This technique is good for headache and nasal
congestion.

Hold the scarf around the bottom of the
receiver's cranium, put your right thumb on the
center of her forehead, and keep your left leg
raised. Next, lean to your right at a 45-degree
angle. Don't bend your arms or use your muscles;
if you want to stretch more, lower your right hip.
Toward the end of the stretch, press her forehead
with your thumb.

Now, switch hand and leg positions and repeat
for the left side.

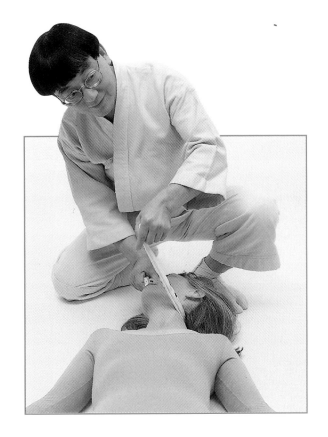

FROM FACE-UP TO FACE-DOWN

After I finish working on the neck, I turn the receiver over in order to work on the back. As in all of Ohashiatsu, it is important to make this change smoothly and with as few movements as possible—be natural, be continuous. I use the receiver's own body weight to move her; I surrender to her, so I don't have to struggle and sweat. Even the biggest bodies can seem weightless when you have mastered the techniques for changing positions.

I usually change the receiver to the face-down position after I have worked on him or her in the face-up position. But if you have a receiver who is very shy or nervous, or simply tired and feeling unsociable, you may want to begin with her face-down. It is a comfortable, nonconfrontational position; you will find that even those who seem unwilling to talk at first will gradually open up as you work on them face-down. Some may get so relaxed that they fall asleep. If they do, continue the session—they will benefit all the same.

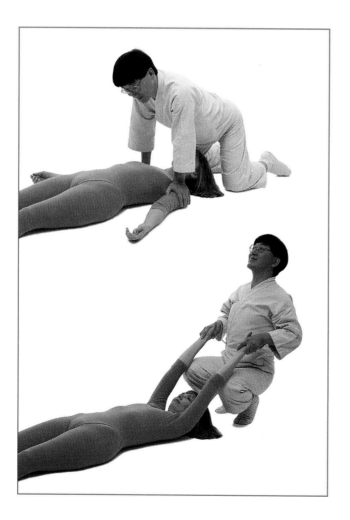

After you have done the last technique on the neck, sit in seiza position and put your hands once more over the receiver's eyes and rest for several seconds, as you did before you started working on the neck. When her eyelashes stop moving, assume a kneeling position and begin to move your hands down her arms to her elbows. Grasp her elbows and lift her arms back over her head. As you do so, raise your knees off the floor and assume a squatting position.

Next, bring the back of her arms over your knees, sliding your hands to her wrists, and stretch her arms by lowering your hips. Release and stretch a couple of times.

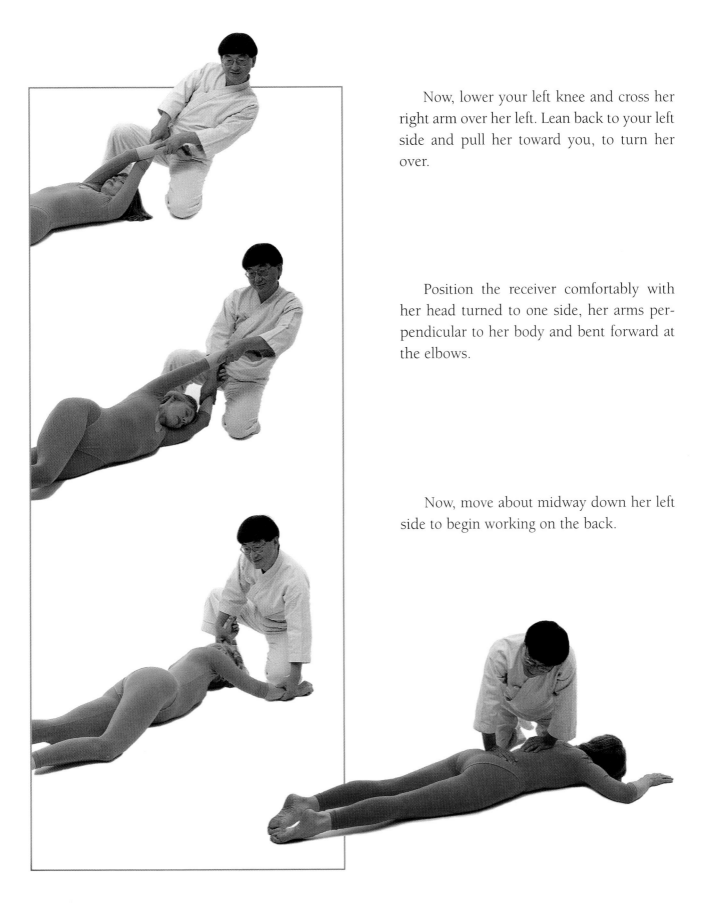

Now, lower your left knee and cross her right arm over her left. Lean back to your left side and pull her toward you, to turn her over.

Position the receiver comfortably with her head turned to one side, her arms perpendicular to her body and bent forward at the elbows.

Now, move about midway down her left side to begin working on the back.

LEANING ON THE BACK

The main meridian on the back of the body is the Bladder meridian, a yang meridian that runs in two parallel lines down each side of the spine (see the meridian charts, page 4). All the techniques in this section work along that meridian. Usually, I work both sides of the spine from the left side of the receiver. But if the receiver is too big for me to reach both sides, I move around to work on the right side.

The back is an area that can store much tension, but it can also tolerate more pressure than other areas. When I work on the back, I sometimes use my elbows in addition to my palms and thumbs, to allow for deeper penetration. I have included the elbow techniques here.

◆ Using your palm and thumb

On the Bladder Meridian
Crossing your arms

◆ Using your elbows

One elbow on the Bladder meridian
Two elbows on the Bladder meridian

USING YOUR PALM AND THUMB

On the Bladder Meridian

To start working on the back, you should be in a crawling position perpendicular to the left side of the receiver's body, with your palms along the two branches of the Bladder meridian on the right side of her spine (see the meridian charts, page 4). Synchronize your breathing with hers.

In the configuration shown here, you apply your right palm to her sacrum, the area at the base of her spine, around Bladder meridian tsubos #25 and #26, and squeeze slightly. Apply your left palm between the upper part of her right shoulder blade and her spine along the meridian line, around the area of Bladder meridian tsubo #12 or #13. Your right hand is the mother hand; your left hand is the messenger hand. Keep both arms

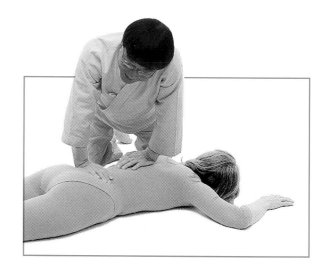

straight, but be in tonus and lean from your hara.

When the receiver is breathing out, bring your hara toward your messenger hand for about five to seven seconds. When she starts breathing in, lean back from your hara and move your messenger hand to the area of Bladder meridian tsubos #14 and #15, supporting your weight with the mother hand and mother knee. Continue along the meridian, leaning in for five to seven seconds at each major tsubo and moving your hara in a figure 8 pattern, until you reach the area of Bladder #22 or #23, just above your mother hand.

Remember to move your right knee when you move your left hand; your left knee is the mother knee and should not move.

Once you have worked the Bladder meridian on the right side of her spine with your left palm, you may repeat with your left thumb. Next, work the meridian on the left side of her spine with palm and then thumb.

Note: If the receiver is too big for you to reach both sides of the spine from his or her left side, work the nearer side first and then use the crossing arms technique (see next page) to move to the other side. (I recommend that you crawl around his head while stretching the back.)

THE BEGINNER'S CRAWL

If you are just beginning to practice Ohashiatsu, I recommend that you crawl at least three times around the receiver before you place your hands on her back (see "Crawling Exercise" in Chapter 2). This will help you to stay in tonus and to remember the importance of cross-patterning.

Whether you are crawling on the floor or working on a human body, maintain the exact same position and attitude. Keeping your back straight and your legs parallel, and having the same distance between hands and knees are all important. Don't tense up when you move from the floor to the body; rather, feel the body as part of the floor. Effortless and natural movement with a relaxed but straight spine will allow you to give efficient Ohashiatsu without any fatigue or injury to yourself or the receiver.

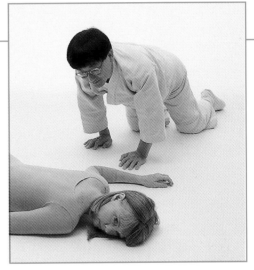

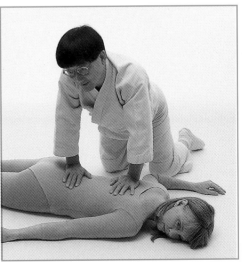

⊘ DON'T!

Because I am sitting back on my legs with my arms bent and my back rounded and tense, I can't move from my hara when working on the Bladder meridian. No matter how hard I press, the pressure will not be effective.

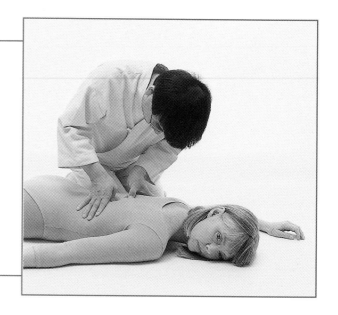

Crossing your arms

This is a useful technique for warming up the back and for moving from one side of the receiver to the other when her back is too big to work on easily from one side.

Cross your arms and apply two palms diagonally on the back, on either side of the spine. When she is breathing out, bring your hara toward her in a circular movement and distribute your body weight evenly.

This stretching technique, like the arm and leg rotations earlier, also gives you the opportunity to move into a new position if you need to, maintaining continuity without disturbing the receiver.

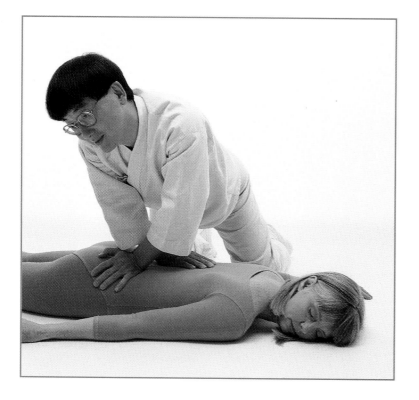

USING YOUR ELBOWS

These techniques take more time than using your palms or thumbs, but they give you a chance to slow down a little during a session, and the receiver usually likes the feeling of deeper penetration.

One elbow on the Bladder meridian

When you use your elbow, your basic movement is the same as when you use your hand. You should still be in a crawling position at the receiver's side. Your right hand (the mother hand) remains on the sacrum, to balance the pressure from your elbow.

Place your left elbow between the upper part of her right shoulder blade and her spine, in the area of Bladder tsubo #12 or #13. Your forearm should be open and relaxed, palm up, at about a 90-degree angle. Squeeze your mother hand and shift your hara toward your elbow. Stay for a few seconds, then lean back toward your mother hand to release, and move your elbow to the next tsubo. Continue working along the meridian, moving

your hara in a figure 8 as you apply and release pressure until you reach the area of Bladder #22 or #23. If you want to go even deeper at any point, slowly bring your left palm toward your left shoulder to "sharpen" your elbow—that is, change the degree of the angle and pressure.

Be sure to pay attention to the mother hand throughout. If you feel the receiver's lower back tensing, you may be applying too much pressure with the elbow—in which case you should release the messenger elbow a little and squeeze the lower back with the mother hand, to dissipate the pain. Then you can try again.

Repeat on the left side of the spine.

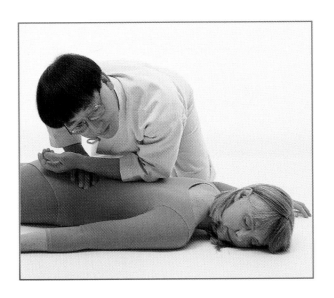

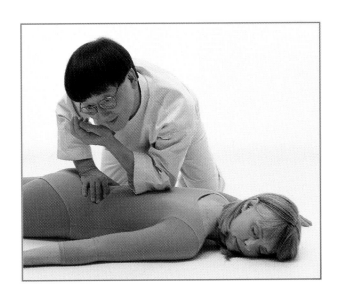

Two elbows on the Bladder meridian

You should still be in the crawling position, but on both of your elbows instead of your palms. Place your right elbow (the mother elbow) on the receiver's sacrum. Put your left elbow on the Bladder meridian between her upper right shoulder blade and her spine, in the area of Bladder meridian tsubos #12 and #13. Both forearms should be open to about a 90-degree angle, palms up. Don't press the bone, and don't let your elbow slip—that can be shocking and irritating for the receiver.

When she breathes out, shift your weight to your right (mother) elbow, and then slowly lean toward your left (messenger) elbow. If the receiver tenses, move your hara back to the mother elbow and wait; then lean again toward

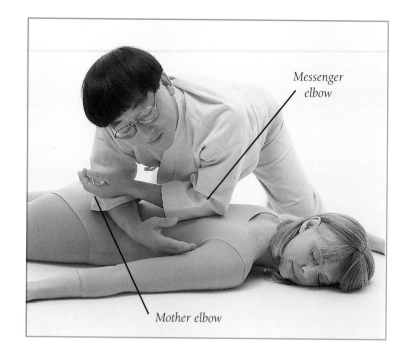

Messenger elbow

Mother elbow

the messenger elbow. After shifting between the two elbows, bring your weight back to the center so that it is equally distributed between both.

Now slowly sharpen your messenger elbow by raising your forearm toward your shoulder. If the receiver tenses up, shift your weight back toward the mother elbow, which is still in the softer position. If the receiver needs more penetration instead, slowly move your right knee (messenger knee) away from her body and lower your hara. Remember that you use your body weight to achieve deeper penetration.

As you did with your palm and thumb, continue along the meridian until you reach Bladder meridian #22 or #23. Lean into each tsubo several seconds.

Repeat on the left side of the spine.

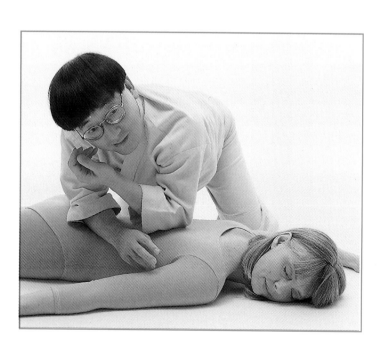

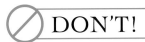

DON'T!

TECHNIQUES TO AVOID USING ON THE BACK

Some practitioners use techniques that they think will display their talents, techniques that may appear more dramatic and complicated than the ones I am showing you. But I find that what seem to be simple and subtle techniques are, in fact, usually more difficult to master—as well as safer and more effective.

In Ohashiatsu, we emphasize that both the giver and receiver should be natural and in tonus. The techniques we use are noninvasive. If you as the giver listen carefully with your mother hand, you will know what is safe and appropriate for the receiver.

The following are examples of techniques that should be avoided because they are either unsafe or ineffective—or both.

When Americans hear about shiatsu, they often ask about walking on the back. I have tried the foot technique myself and even included an example of it in my first book. But from my 25 years of experience, and from speaking with other practitioners and with my clients, I have concluded that the foot is not as effective as some believe.

You cannot use your mother hand when you are standing on the receiver's back, and the foot itself is not sensitive enough to tell you how the receiver is reacting. If you try standing on the back with two feet, you may not only be applying far too much body weight; you may also have trouble keeping your balance. You cannot maintain tonicity or continuity if you are struggling just to remain upright—and you could do considerable damage to yourself and the receiver by falling from this position! So, in the end, I think it is better not to walk on the back.

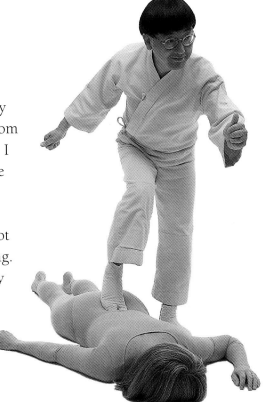

⊘ **DON'T!**

Some givers try to stretch the back by stepping on the spine and pulling back the arms. This is a dangerous technique that could dislocate the receiver's shoulder or injure the spine, and it also strains the giver.

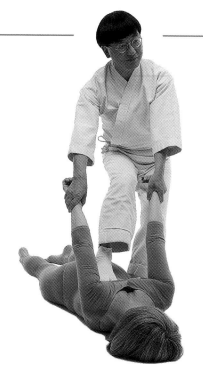

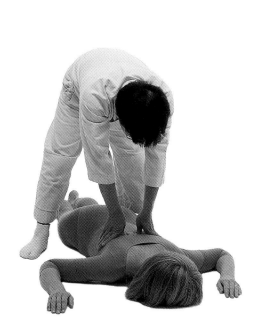

I don't understand why some givers stand over the receiver with their backs rounded. This bad habit guarantees maximum fatigue for the giver and minimum benefit for the receiver.

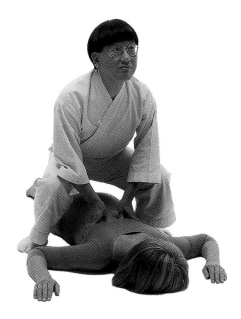

The same is true when the giver squats over the receiver. Here the giver's movement is homologous and can feel abrupt to the receiver.

DANCING ALONG THE LEGS AND LOWER BACK

Sequence

- ◆ Using your palm and thumb

    On the Bladder meridian, upper leg

    On the Bladder meridian, lower leg

    From one leg to the other

- ◆ Using your knees

    One knee on the Bladder meridian, upper leg

    Two knees on the Bladder meridian, upper leg

    From one leg to the other

From the outside to the inside of the leg

    One knee on the Kidney and Liver meridians, upper leg

    Two knees on the Kidney and Liver meridians, upper leg

    Working the lower back

From the lower back to the right leg

When you work on the legs in the face-down position, you will be working on the Bladder meridian, a yang meridian that runs in two branches down the back of the upper legs to the knee and then in a single branch down the calf to the foot, and the Kidney and Liver meridians, yin meridians that run up the inside of the legs (see the meridian charts, pages 4, 5, and 6). First, learn to work on these meridians with your palm and thumb. Only after you have mastered those techniques should you try the knee techniques presented in this section.

Knee techniques are extremely powerful. They allow you to give more pressure—and to assume a different posture, which can add variety and prevent fatigue—but they also require greater flexibility and balance on the part of the giver. So, practice with your knees only after you feel confident about using your palm and thumb. When using your knees, be sure to ask the receiver if he or she experiences any discomfort.

USING YOUR PALM AND THUMB

On the Bladder meridian, upper leg

After you finish working on the back, remain in the crawling position and move slightly down the left side of the receiver to begin working on the left leg. Put your left (mother) hand on her sacrum in the area of Bladder tsubos #25 and #26 (see the meridian charts, page 4). Put your right (messenger) hand on Bladder tsubo #36, just below the buttock. Next, palm down the back of the leg to the back of the kneecap (Bladder #40) two or three times, moving your hara in a figure 8 and leaning into the major tsubos along the way. As you do so, squeeze the sacrum with your mother hand.

Now, go down the meridian with your thumb two or three times. Never press hard on the back of the kneecap. Be sure to keep your knees open and your toes relaxed. Remember cross-patterning.

After you have used your palm and your thumb, grasp the back of the kneecap with your right hand, which now becomes your mother hand. With your left hand, thumb down the meridian once while your right hand squeezes the back of the kneecap. As you do so, crawl sideways to your right, so that you are facing her lower leg. Now, you are in position to work the Bladder meridian in the lower leg.

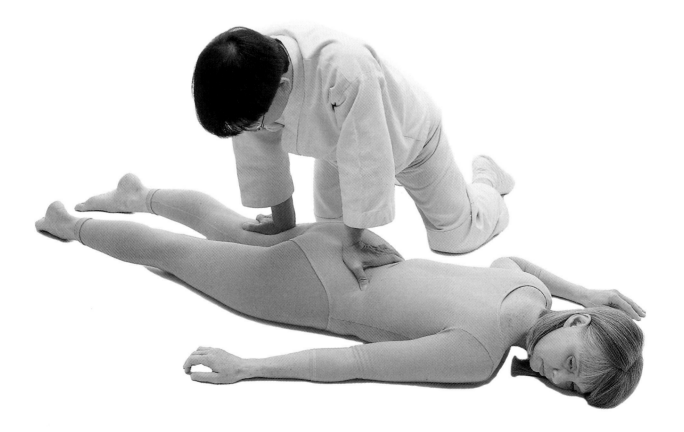

On the Bladder meridian, lower leg

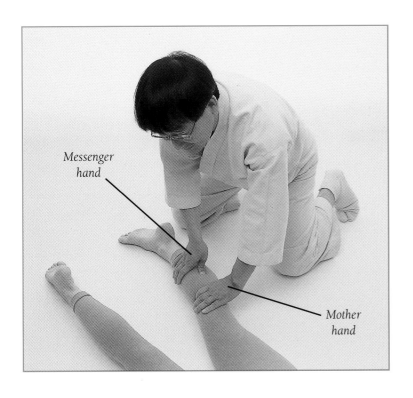

Messenger hand

Mother hand

Your left hand now becomes the mother hand, squeezing the back of the kneecap in the area of Bladder tsubo #40. With your right (messenger) hand, palm down the Bladder meridian along the middle of the calf in the lower leg to Bladder #60 in the area between the outside edge of the anklebone and the Achilles tendon. Repeat two or three times with the palm, then two or three times with the thumb. Always listen with your mother hand; abrupt pressure may cause a spasm in the receiver's leg. If you are not sure of her reaction, ask whether she feels any pain.

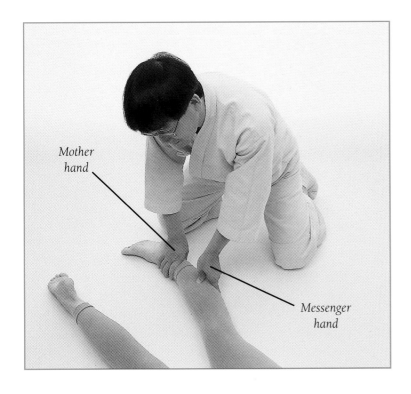

Mother hand

Messenger hand

After you have gone down the meridian with your palm and thumb, grasp her ankle with your right hand, which now becomes the mother hand. Next, thumb down the meridian once with your left hand; don't forget to move your right knee as you go. Now, you are ready to make the transition to the right leg.

From one leg to the other

After you have finished working the Bladder meridian in the left lower leg, grasp her left ankle with your left hand. Crawl around so that you are facing the receiver's feet and grasp her right ankle with your right hand.

Next, cross the toes of her left foot over the toes of her right foot, and hold both firmly with your left hand. Release your right hand and place it on her sacrum. Now, bend her legs toward her buttocks and while they are bent, move your body around to about midway up her right side.

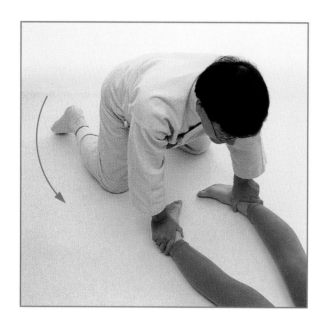

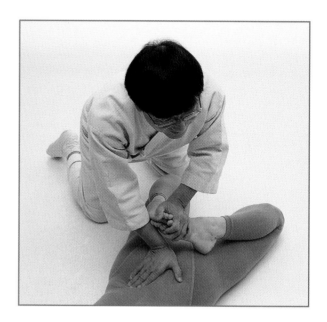

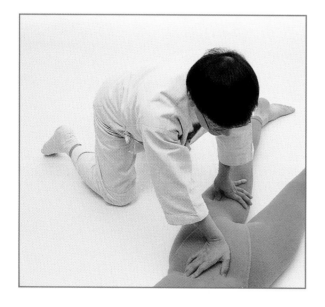

Lower her legs to the floor. Keep your right (mother) hand in place on the sacrum, and put your left (messenger) hand at Bladder tsubo #36, just below the right buttock. Now, you are ready to begin working the Bladder meridian in the upper right leg.

Note: You may modify the above transition so that you can also work on the Kidney and Liver meridians on the inner left leg (see note, page 112) and on the Bladder meridian in the lower back (see note, page 113).

USING YOUR KNEES

One knee on the Bladder meridian, upper leg

Put your left hand on the receiver's sacrum in the area of Bladder tsubos #25 and #26 (see the meridian charts, page 4). With your right hand, grasp the back of her kneecap, around Bladder #40. Next, place your left knee on her Bladder meridian just below the buttock, in the area of Bladder #36. When she breathes out, lean toward her and turn her leg toward your knee; raise your hips and squeeze with both hands. When she breathes in, release the pressure and move your knee down to the next major tsubo. Continue down the meridian to her knee, holding for about three to five seconds at each major tsubo. Repeat two or three times.

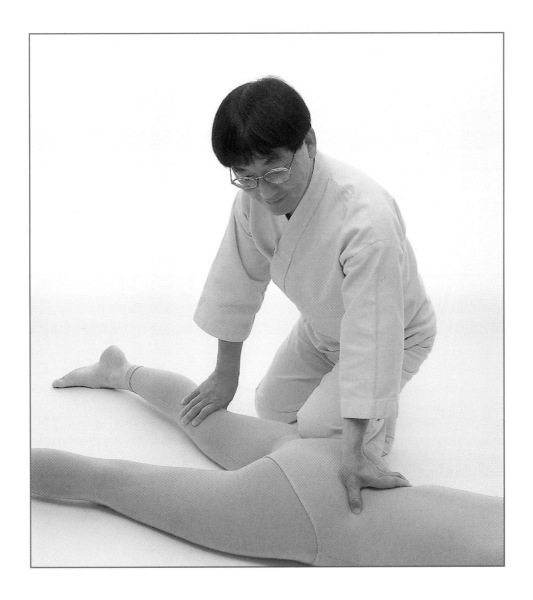

Two knees on the Bladder meridian, upper leg

If you are especially flexible and the receiver can tolerate more pressure, this is a stronger technique to use on the back of the upper leg.

Assume a squatting position, with your left hand still on the receiver's sacrum and your right hand still holding the back of her kneecap. Next, turn the receiver's leg toward you and bring your knees to her Bladder meridian, with your left knee just below her buttock (around Bladder #36) and move your right knee close beside it (be careful not to hit the bone). Keep your body weight balanced on your toes.

Now, move your knees, one after the other, bit by bit down the meridian. To increase pressure, raise your hips. If she feels pain, squeeze with both hands and release pressure from your knees.

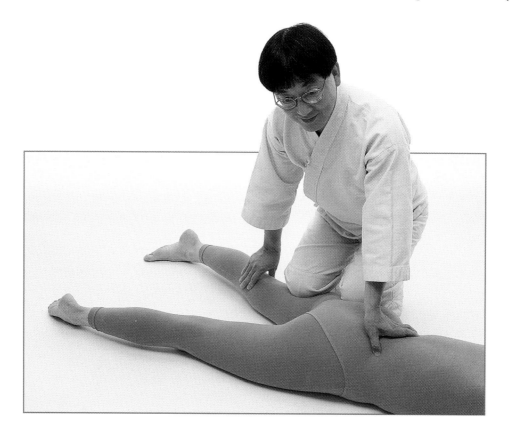

From One Leg to the Other

As you make this transition, you also work on the Kidney and Liver (yin) meridians on the inner legs and the Bladder (yang) meridian in the lower back. In the pages that follow, each stage of the transition is presented as a separate technique, but in practice they should all flow together.

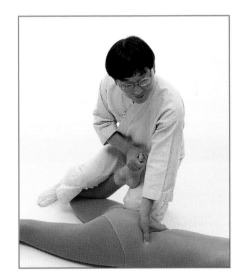

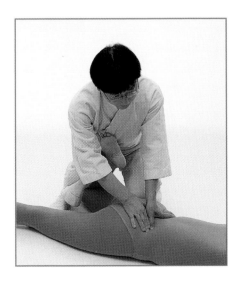

From the outside to the inside of the leg

After you have finished working the Bladder meridian in the lower leg with your palm and thumb, place both of your knees on the receiver's upper leg, so that your left knee is just below the buttock (Bladder #36) and your right knee is around the middle of the thigh, in the area of Bladder #37. Keep your left hand on her sacrum.

Next, pick up her leg by holding her foot with your right hand and bend it toward you; raise your hips to increase the pressure of your knees, and squeeze both hands.

Now, lower your hips, remove your right knee, and bend her leg further toward her back. Bring your right leg in to her shinbone, to keep her leg bent. Bring your right hand to her sacrum, beside your left hand, and squeeze with both hands.

Now, remove your left knee, grasp her left foot with your left hand and move her left leg out to the side, at the same time moving your body in between her legs and putting your right knee near her kneecap in the area of Kidney tsubo #10 (see the meridian charts, page 5).

Note: You may also perform this transition without using your knees, in order to get into position to work the Kidney and Liver meridians with your palm or thumb. If you are going to do so, you will lower the receiver's left leg to the floor as you move your body in between her legs (see the previous step). Then you will use your left hand to work the meridians.

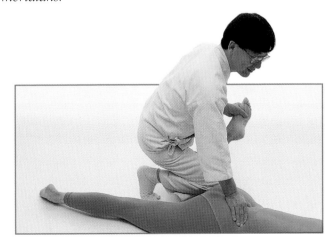

One knee on the Kidney and Liver meridians, upper leg

Work the Kidney meridian in the upper left leg with your right knee, starting just above Kidney tsubo #10 (see the meridian charts, page 5). Lean into the meridian as you move your knee, until you reach the upper thigh. Repeat several times.

Now, push her left foot out a little further to the side, to expose the Liver meridian, and work up that meridian with your right knee several times from Liver tsubo #8 to #10.

Note: You may also work the meridians with your left palm or thumb.

Two knees on the Kidney and Liver meridians, upper leg

After you have worked the Kidney and Liver meridians with one knee, remove that knee, lower the receiver's leg to the floor, and put your left hand on the back of her kneecap (your right hand remains on her sacrum). You are still in between her legs, facing her head.

Next, turn your body so that you are perpendicular to the Kidney meridian on her left leg, squat, and bring both knees into the meridian, so that your left knee is just above her kneecap (Kidney #10) and your right knee is beside your left one.

Work up the meridian in the leg, alternating knees. First, lean into your right knee; then lean back to release pressure, and lean into your left. As you are leaning toward your left knee, move your right knee to the next major tsubo on the meridian. Next, lean toward the right and move your left knee—and so on, until your right knee reaches the top of the inner thigh and your left knee is just beside it. Raise and lower your hips to keep your body weight comfortably distributed,

and move your hara in a figure 8 . If the receiver expresses discomfort, squeeze both hands and release the pressure from your knees.

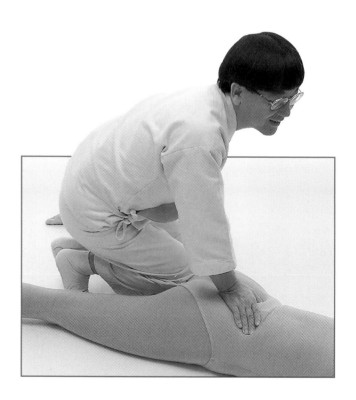

Working the lower back

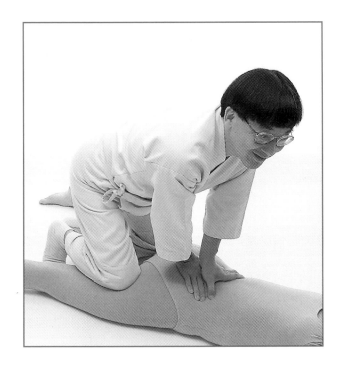

Remove your knees from the receiver and turn your body so that you face her head. Place both hands on her sacrum. Next, put your right knee on her right leg and your left knee on her left leg, on the Bladder meridian in the area of tsubo #36 (see the meridian charts, page 4), just below the buttocks. Move your hara in a figure 8.

Now, open your hands and use your thumbs to work on the Bladder meridian in the lower back, in the area of Bladder #23; equalize the pressure of your hands and knees.

Note: You may, of course, work on the lower back with your knees on the floor, rather than on the receiver's legs. Sometimes, if I want deeper penetration, I use my elbows on the lower back—but with extreme caution, never touching the spine.

From the lower back to the right leg

After you have finished working on the lower back, turn to your right and move your left knee onto her right leg next to your right knee.

Now slide your right knee off her leg onto the floor, pick up her right foot with your right hand, and bend her leg toward her buttocks at about a 45-degree angle.

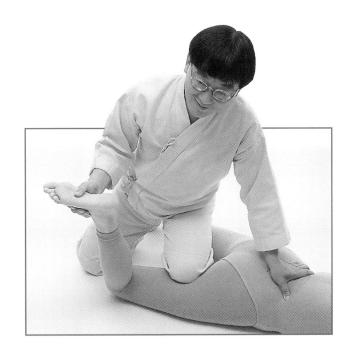

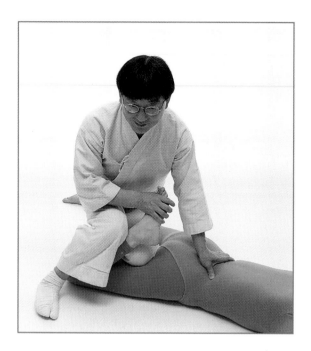

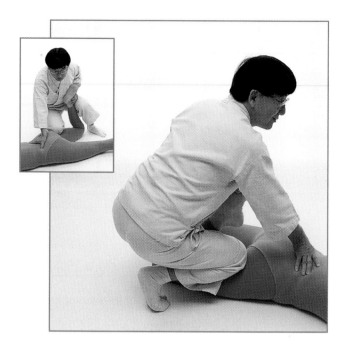

Bring your right knee around to keep her leg bent; then release your right hand from her foot and put it on her sacrum beside your left.

Now lift your left knee off her leg, release your left hand from her sacrum, and grasp her foot while you bring your right knee further around the outside of her right leg, and place it just below her buttock.

Then bring your left knee around and place it on the floor perpendicular to her right leg. Lower her leg and place your left hand just below the back of the kneecap. With your right knee work the Bladder meridian in her upper leg two or three times.

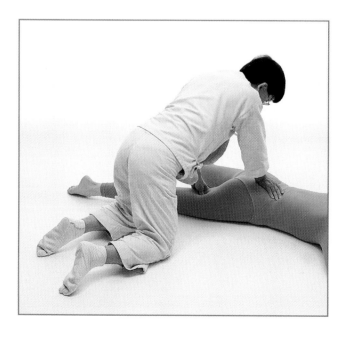

Now slide your right knee onto the floor beside your left so that you are in a crawling position, ready to repeat all the techniques of this section (palm, thumb, and knees) on her right leg, switching hands and knees accordingly.

FROM FACE-DOWN TO FACE-UP

1

After you have finished working on the receiver's right leg in the face-down position, grasp both of her feet with your left hand, bend her legs back toward her buttocks and move around her knees toward her left side.

About halfway around, switch hands, so that your right hand is holding her feet and your left hand is on her sacrum.

2

When you are midway up her left side, gently lower her legs to the floor, place your right hand on her sacrum and with your left hand bring her right arm onto the floor above her head.

Now (again with your left hand) grasp her elbow and bring her left arm across her back, palm up and bent at the elbow. Use your right knee to hold her elbow in place while you slide your left hand up her spine, along the Governing Vessel meridian (see the meridian charts, page 7), and take hold of the front of the left shoulder.

3

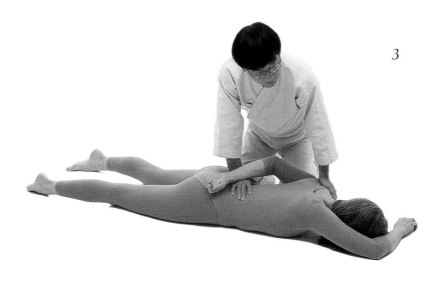

Next, slide your right hand down her left leg to her foot, pick it up and bend her leg so that her knee is as close to her chest as possible.

Then, slide your hand up her calf and grasp the back of her kneecap. Now lift her left shoulder with your left hand and turn her face-up. (Be sure she doesn't turn onto her left arm.) As you are doing this, lift her left leg with your right hand and take it in the same direction as her shoulder.

4

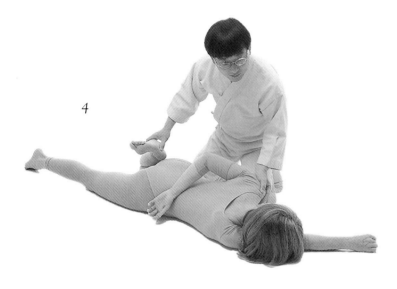

5

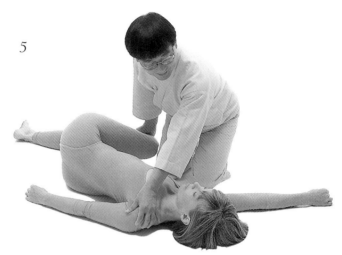

Then, slide the side of your left hand down the center of her chest, along the Conception Vessel meridian, to her hara. When the receiver is fully face-up, turn to face her head, bring your right hand around to the front of her kneecap, and rotate her leg several times.

Then lower it to the floor, place your right hand on her hara beside your left, and repeat the hara diagnosis.

6

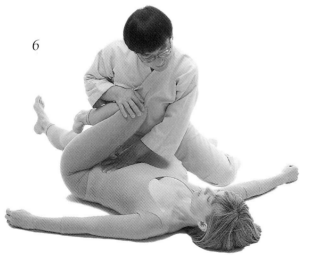

7

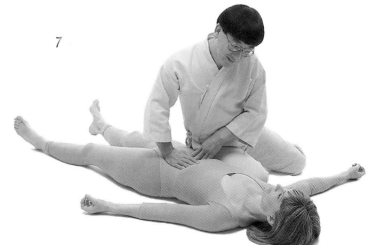

CRADLING THE HEAD

The face and head are extremely yang parts of the body—usually warm, active, and volatile. The face is delicate and sensitive, and like the neck and hara, you have to approach working on the face with special respect and awareness. If you don't feel comfortable, neither will the receiver. It is hard to give a session on the face and head because not only is it a small area, but it is also a complicated one: There are about 50 to 60 small muscles in the face alone. I recommend that you move your hands and fingers slowly. Take your time—follow the receiver's response rather than your own style. Moving from your hara may be more difficult because of the restricted area you are working on, but it is still possible—and when you move from your hara, your touch will feel much better to the receiver than if you were using tense fingertips.

Usually, I work on the face and head at the end of a session, when the receiver is feeling more relaxed and accepting. When I give Ohashiatsu to this part of the body, I feel honored to know that I am respected and trusted. I sense that the receiver has surrendered to me, and this makes me feel maternal—my ki energy springs forth without any effort.

Use as few or as many of these techniques as you have time for—or that you feel are appropriate for the receiver. The sequence itself can be very flexible. Here, I have grouped them according to the part of the face, working down from the forehead, out to the temples, and ending at the ears.

From the hara to the face and head

This is the same transition you use when you move from the hara to work on the arms (see page 71).

Slide the side of your right hand up along the Conception Vessel meridian, in the center of the chest and over, to take hold of her right shoulder.

Next, slide the side of your left hand up the meridian, over your right hand, and take hold of her left shoulder.

Now, lean toward her, raise your hips, and move around behind her head so that you are centered between her shoulders.

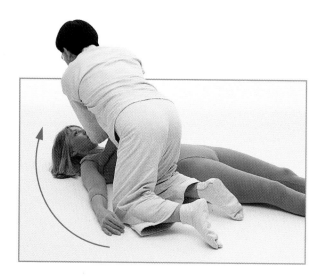 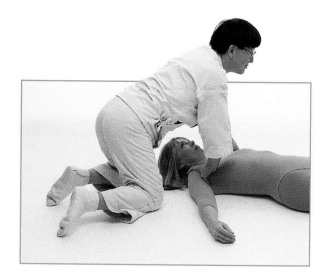

Preparation

Nobody wants to be touched on the face if he or she does not like or trust you, so always appreciate the fact that a receiver is allowing you to do so: it means that you are respected and loved. So, calm yourself before you begin by meditating for a couple of minutes. (You may even gasho again, if you like.)

Rub down your hands for two or three minutes to make them warm. If they (or the receiver's face) are sweaty or oily, you can use a light cotton, rectangular scarf and administer the techniques through it. I recommend the same if your hands

are cold (although they probably won't be this late in a session).

You will work mostly from a squatting position behind the receiver's head. Keep one knee raised, for balance and flexibility. It does not matter which knee, but if you are right-handed, it will be most natural to raise your left knee.

Note: If the receiver is wearing contact lenses, don't do any techniques on the eyelids or close to the eyes.

From the forehead up

This technique is good for headache, eye tension, and insomnia.

Position yourself comfortably behind the receiver's head, allowing enough room for you to move from your hara. Place both your thumbs on the center of her forehead, side by side, just above her eyebrows (your fingers rest lightly on the temples). When she breathes out, lean toward her head and press firmly. Don't tense your thumbs; just bring your hara to them. When she breathes in, release the pressure and move your thumbs an inch or so apart, toward the temples. Press again, release again, and continue moving your thumbs inch by inch until you reach the temples.

Then return to the center of the forehead, a little higher up than before, and repeat. Move higher again, and repeat again. Depending on the height of the forehead, you should move across it with your thumbs three or four times, up to the hairline. You can also do this technique with four fingers of each hand, instead of the thumbs, for a different feeling.

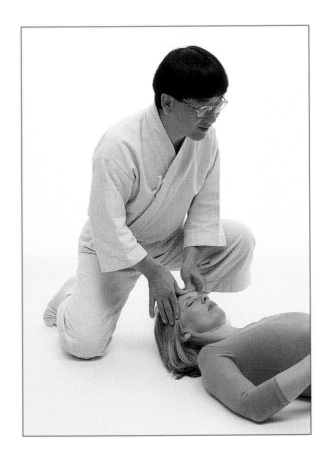

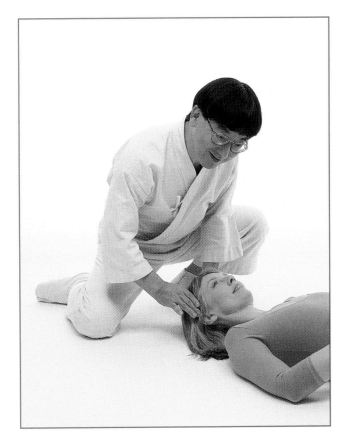

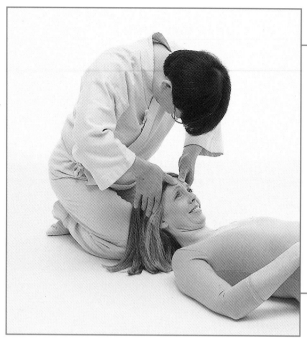

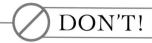

When you are working on the head, face, and neck areas, don't put the receiver's head on your lap: It will be uncomfortable for the receiver, and it will be difficult for you to use your entire body. It limits your flexibility and hara movement, forcing you to bend your back in an awkward way and to tense your hands.

Palms over eyes

After you finish each technique, apply both of your palms to the receiver's eyes and rest for a few seconds, just as you did when you were working on the neck. If she is relaxed and comfortable, her eyelashes will move very little and you can continue on to the next technique. If her lashes are moving fairly vigorously, give her more time to relax by keeping your palms on her eyes longer. Doing this can slow down her heartbeat and also give you time to rest. Don't apply your hands suddenly, and never press.

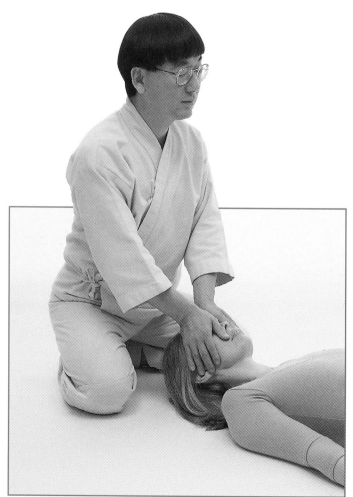

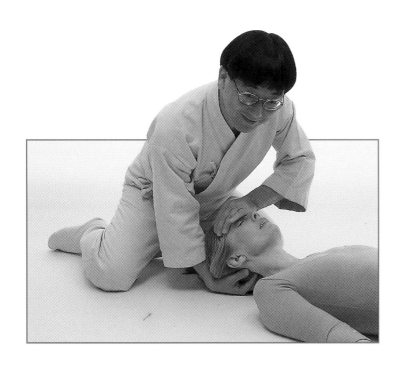

Forehead and neck

This is a great technique for relaxing the entire body, including the spine, hips, and legs.

Apply your left hand to the center of the receiver's forehead and your right hand to the back of her head, where it dips. When she breathes out, slide both hands slowly toward you, gently pulling her neck, and move your hara down. Repeat a few times.

THE EYES

Eye sockets

The points around the eye socket are useful for treating eye problems, fatigue, nasal and sinus congestion, headache, and even insomnia.

Apply both of your thumbs or little fingers to Bladder tsubo #1 at the inner corners of the eye sockets, which we call the *sei mei* (bright light) point (see the meridian charts, page 4). Don't press; rather, pull: The movement is inward and then outward, as if you were scooping toward yourself. Repeat several times.

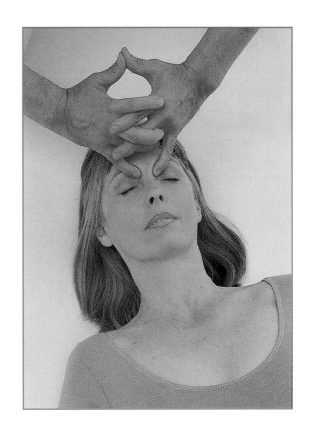

Eyelids

This is good for nervous people and emotional situations.

Apply four fingers of each hand to the receiver's eyelids. When she is breathing out, vibrate your fingers gently. When she is breathing in, stop vibrating. Repeat the procedure several times.

For variety, you may use your thumbs instead.

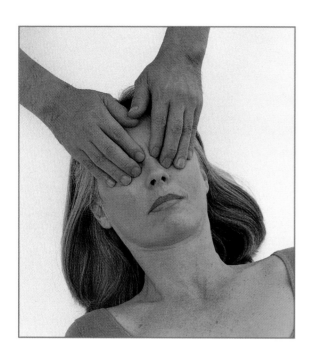

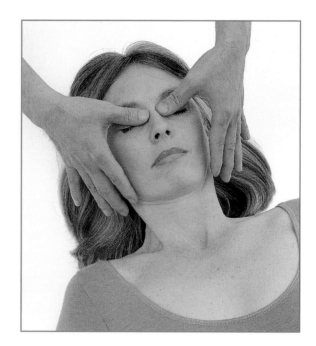

Eyebrows

This technique is good for tired eyes.

Apply either four fingers or the thumb of both hands just under the receiver's eyebrows and pull up. Don't press the eyeballs; gently pull the eyebrow upward toward you. Repeat when she is breathing out.

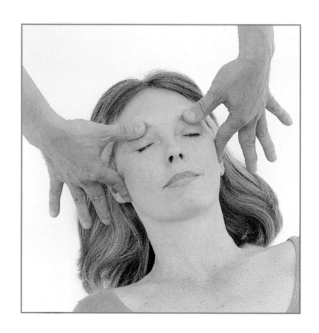

THE NOSE AND SINUSES

Nostrils

This relieves nasal congestion.

Apply either your thumb, middle finger, or little finger to the edge of the receiver's nostril at Large Intestine #20 (see the meridian charts, page 2). The traditional name for this point is *welcome smell,* and that is its function: to activate the sense of smell. Press several times while she is breathing out. Then repeat on the other nostril.

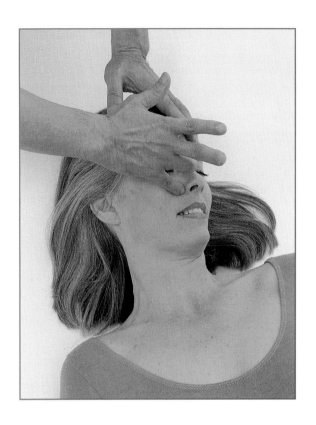

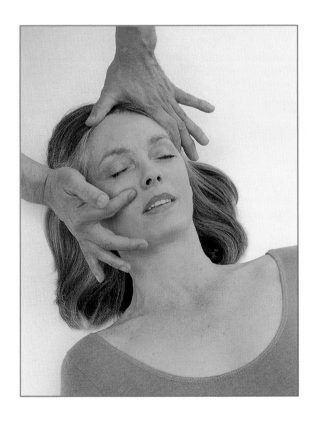

Cheekbones

This is also good for nasal and sinus congestion. The point will be especially sensitive if the condition is advanced.

Turn the receiver's face about 45 degrees to one side. Apply your index finger to approximately the center of her cheekbone, just below the eye. To keep your finger from slipping off, press very slowly. As an extra precaution, you can cover her eye with the palm of your other hand. Press up toward yourself, not down toward the teeth. Repeat several times. Then turn her face and work on the other cheekbone.

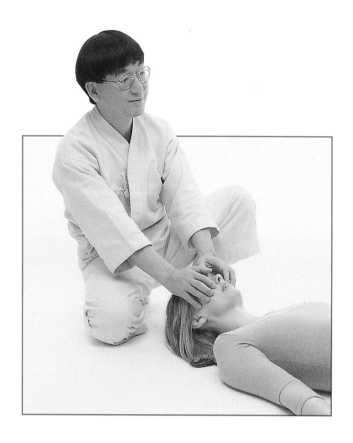

Stronger cheekbone technique

Apply four fingers of each hand to the receiver's cheekbones. When she exhales, squeeze upward toward yourself, and hold for three to five seconds. When she inhales, relax your fingers and move them a little further toward the temples, then repeat. Move and repeat at about three places along the cheekbones until you reach the temples.

THE TEMPLES

With palms

Many people have lots of tension in the temple area because of jaw, neck, or lower back pain, nasal congestion, or headache.

First, apply the heels of your palms to her temples. When she exhales, slowly squeeze her head at the temple. Hold for five to seven seconds. Release when she inhales. Repeat several times. I occasionally vibrate my palms while I am squeezing.

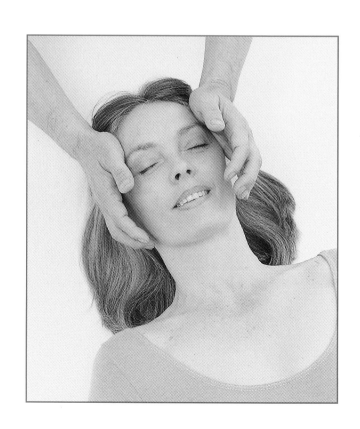

With two thumbs

For stronger pressure on the temples, try this technique.

Apply both thumbs to the temples, and the fingers of each hand to the back of the head just behind the ears. Gently squeeze both thumbs and fingers, distributing the pressure evenly. While the receiver is breathing out, slowly pull her head toward you and vibrate slightly. She should open her mouth and surrender to this technique.

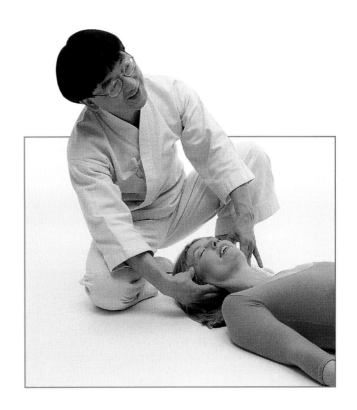

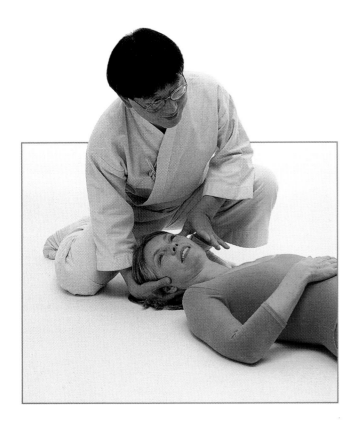

With one thumb

If the receiver is too sensitive for the previous technique, you can do one temple at a time.

Hold the back of her head with your right palm, and turn her face 45 degrees to the right. Put your left thumb on her left temple and slowly lean in, to apply pressure when she exhales. If she feels pain, squeeze the fingers of your right hand. Repeat several times.

Then, turn her head to the other side, switch hands, and repeat for the right temple.

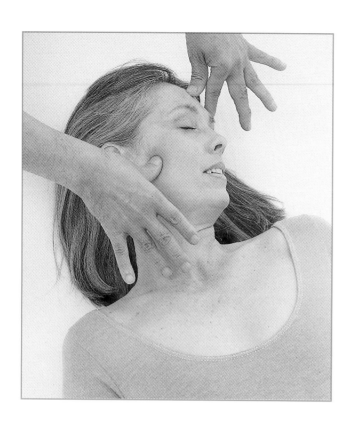

THE JAWBONE

This technique is good for easing tension in the jaw.

Apply your thumb to the jawbone in front of the ear, in the area of Small Intestine #19 (see the meridian charts, page 3). Her jaw should be open and relaxed. Gently press and move your thumb in a circle, to move her jaw. For variety, you can also use your little finger or index finger on this point.

THE EARS

The ears are very sensitive, yet touch is very soothing to them. If you give good technique to the ear, it is very satisfying to the receiver.

With finger or thumb

Turn the receiver's face to the left and apply your little finger just behind the earlobe. Press gently in a circular motion. Turn her face to the other side and repeat.

You may also use the thumb or index finger on this point.

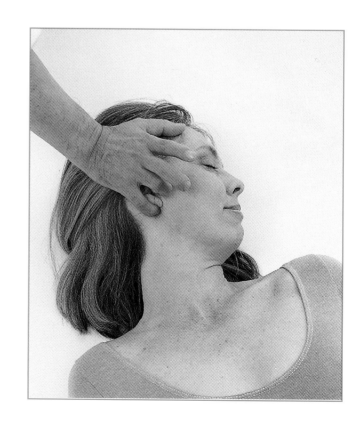

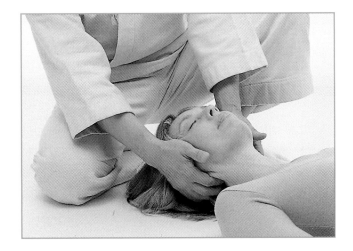

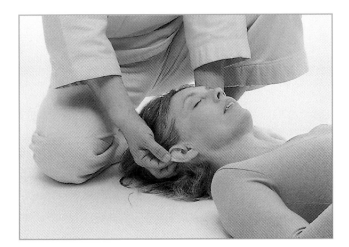

With palms and fingers

This technique is especially relaxing. It is a good one to do at the very end of a face session.

Put your palms over both her ears, sealing off any noise. Hold firmly for five to seven seconds, then gently vibrate. Don't release your hands suddenly—slide them off, since you may have created suction in the ear.

Now, grasp the fleshy part of the ear and the earlobe, squeeze gently between your thumb and index finger, and pull gently away from the face. Go over the ears in this manner a couple of times.

Return from the face and head to the hara

After I finish working on the face and head, I am also usually at the end of the Ohashiatsu session, so I return to the receiver's hara.

Put your palms over the receiver's eyes once more, then slide your hands down her face, cross your left hand over your right one, and place your palms on the top of her shoulders. Lean forward, raise your hips, and crawl around to the receiver's right side to her hara (your arms will naturally uncross as you go), parallel to her body, facing her head. Release your hands from her shoulders and slide them, one by one, down the Conception Vessel meridian to her hara.

Sit in seiza. Synchronize your breathing and meditate for a while. Now, remove both hands from the receiver and perform gasho again.

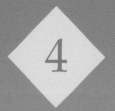

Moving in
Tonus . . .
the Side Position

The side position is extremely comfortable for receivers, especially for those who are tired, overweight, pregnant, have a heart problem (in this case, the left side should be up), or even those who are bedridden. Because contact in this position can be reassuring, I sometimes begin on the side with people who are receiving Ohashiatsu for the first time. Apart from the special needs it can meet, this is the only position that allows access to the Gall Bladder meridian on the rib cage and hip (see page 140) and an opportunity for a full-body stretch (see page 144).

For the giver, working on a receiver in the side position requires less movement than when the receiver is face-up or face-down; you move only up and down the body (sideways), not around. As a result, however, you need greater flexibility; you will need to move more from your hara and to be especially careful about maintaining your balance and supporting the receiver. You may want to review the kata exercises in Chapter 2 that emphasize these skills before you try the following techniques. The side position is especially useful for teaching you how to bring the receiver's body toward you, to practice pulling, rather than pushing.

In this chapter, as well as the others, there are many different techniques to learn. Remember my advice: Don't try to master them all in one day. And don't try to use them all in a single session. Select only a few techniques each time you work. You will gradually learn which techniques are the best ones to use for a particular person at a particular time, and in accordance with your own skill, development, and movement.

Preparation

Have the receiver lie comfortably on her left side. Her left arm should be relaxed and extended in front of her body. Her right arm should also be extended, but bent slightly at the elbow. Her right leg should be in front of her left, and bent at the knee.

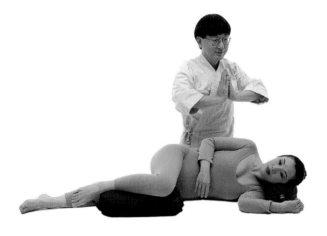

Place a pillow under her neck and her right knee. The pillows must be firm in order to support these areas of the body. I use Japanese-style cylindrical or rectangular pillows made from buckwheat hulls, which are available in the United States from many sources—such as stores that sell futons or through advertisements in health magazines.

Once you have positioned the receiver, sit in seiza behind her, parallel to her body, near her shoulder and facing her head. Perform gashyo, or simply close your eyes for two or three minutes in order to relax and focus yourself.

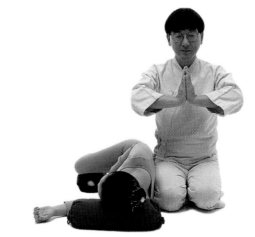

WARMING UP THE HEAD AND SHOULDERS

◆ Shoulder rotation

◆ Working the Gall Bladder meridian

Shoulder rotation

This rotation is a warm-up technique that will tell you how flexible the receiver's shoulder is. The more flexible it is, the more you can stretch it.

Raise your left leg and place her right arm on your right forearm or elbow. Intertwine the fingers of both your hands, and grasp the top of her right shoulder.

WARMING UP THE HEAD AND SHOULDERS

Rotate the shoulder clockwise and then counter-clockwise, three to five times in each direction. Her head should move slightly as you do this. Don't tense your hands and arms; rotate her shoulder by rotating your hara.

Keep your spine straight.

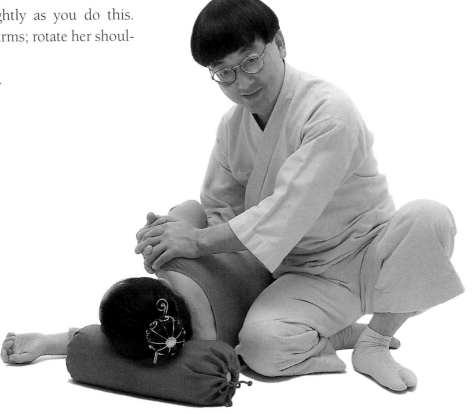

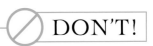 DON'T!

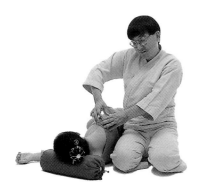

If I don't raise my left leg, I tend to round my shoulders and cannot move with my entire body; I am forced to rely on muscle power and can easily become tired. So, be sure to raise one leg and keep your spine straight.

And because I'm not supporting her arm on my forearm, I don't have a secure grasp of her shoulder. I can't rotate fully, and her arm may flop around.

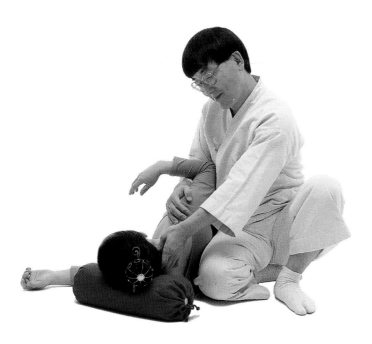

Working the Gall Bladder meridian

After rotating the receiver's shoulder, release your left hand and apply it to the back right side of her neck, as if you were going to squeeze it; your thumb should be in the area of Gall Bladder #20 (see the meridian charts, page 6). Pull her shoulder back toward you, to give a good stretch to the neck.

Next, palm down the neck and out to the middle of the shoulder, in the area of Gall Bladder #21. Repeat two or three times.

Now, place your left palm on her temple, in the area of Gall Bladder #1, and hold while you pull her shoulder toward you in order to stretch more. Remember to use your hara to create the pulling action of your hand.

After you have finished, rotate the shoulder again two or three times.

If you think the receiver can tolerate deeper penetration, you can repeat this technique using your thumb—slowly and carefully.

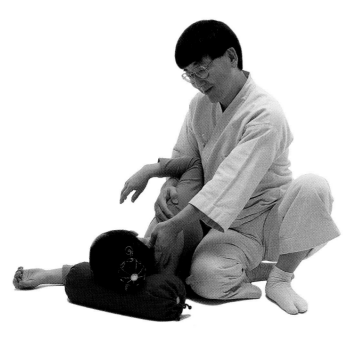

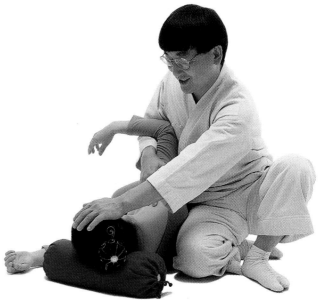

STRETCHING AND PULLING ALONG THE ARMS

Sequence

- ◆ Arm rotation
- ◆ Working the Lung meridian (yin)
- ◆ Working the Heart Constrictor meridian (yin)
- ◆ Working the Heart meridian (yin)

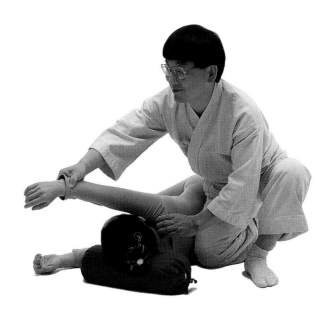

Arm rotation

You will now rotate the arm and move into position to work the Lung meridian. In the side position, you rotate the arm as you go from one meridian to the next. As with the leg rotations in the face-up position, these rotations are not only good exercise and therapy for the receiver, they are also a transitional technique for the giver.

Hold the receiver's right wrist from underneath with your right (messenger) hand. Place the fingers of your left (mother) hand across the top of her shoulder, in the area between the shoulder blade and the spine. Keep your left knee raised and put your left elbow against the inside of it. Supporting your elbow with your knee helps you keep your balance and secures your mother (left) hand—and here the mother hand is most important, because it keeps the receiver's body from slipping backward or forward.

Now, rotate her arm in the widest possible circle, two or three times clockwise and counterclockwise. As you rotate, coordinate your mother hand with your messenger hand; as you bring her arm toward you, your mother hand should press in the opposite direction from the messenger hand, in order to stretch the arm to the fullest extent.

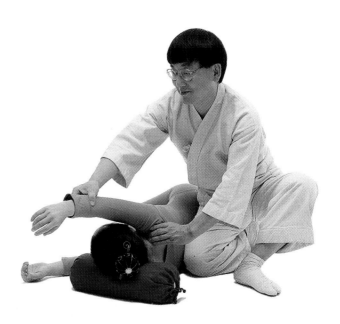

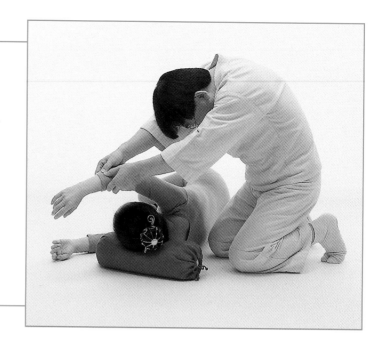

⊘ DON'T!

This is the wrong way to do an arm rotation. I am holding the receiver's arm with both hands, rather than using one hand to support her shoulder. Without the support of my mother hand on her shoulder, I risk losing control of her body. And without my leg raised, I may also lose my balance. I cannot achieve a full rotation and stretch in this position.

Working the Lung meridian (yin)

As you finish rotating the receiver's arm, bring your left knee down and your right knee up, supporting your weight on the toes of both feet (heels raised), as you learned in Chapter 2 (see "Squatting," page 37). Lower her arm, palm up, onto your right knee for support, and with the fingers of your left (mother) hand, hold Lung meridian tsubo #1, about an inch below the middle of the collarbone (see the meridian charts, page 2). Put your right hand beside your left hand.

When she is breathing out, squeeze both hands and stretch her arm by leaning back. Now, release and move your right hand to the next major tsubo. Continue in this way up the meridian along the outer edge of the arm to the thumb, Lung #11. Repeat several times.

Working the Heart Constrictor meridian (yin)

Rotate the receiver's arm again and, as you finish, bring it (extended and palm out) against your chest. If you are small, you may want to keep your left knee raised to give you better balance; otherwise, you can put both knees on the floor.

Slide your right hand down to hold Heart Constrictor tsubo #2, at the outer edge of the armpit (see the meridian charts, page 5), and place your left hand just beside it. Squeeze both hands and *lean back* to stretch her arm. When you give the same amount of pressure with both hands, the receiver feels much less pain and will be able to accept deeper and stronger techniques sooner.

Now, work up the meridian along the middle of the inner arm with your left hand, squeezing and leaning at the major tsubos, until you reach the tip of the middle finger, Heart Constrictor #9.

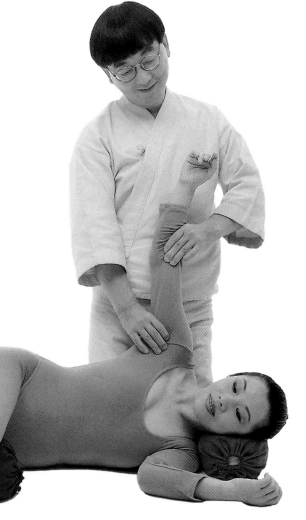

Working the Heart meridian (yin)

As you rotate the receiver's arm raise your left knee to get into position to work the Heart meridian. At the end of the rotation bring the arm down (extended and palm out) to be supported on your raised left knee.

Move your right hand down to hold Heart meridian tsubo #1, at the base of the armpit (see the meridian charts, page 3), and bring your left hand beside it to the meridian at the innermost top of the upper arm. Squeeze with both hands and lean back from your hara.

Lower your left knee to stretch her arm further. Then release, and move your left hand up the meridian, which runs along the innermost edge of the arm, to the next major tsubo. Squeeze again, and lean again. Continue in this manner to tsubo #9 on the inside tip of the little finger.

When you have finished working the meridians in the arm, you will rotate the arm again and get into position to work the Bladder meridian on the back.

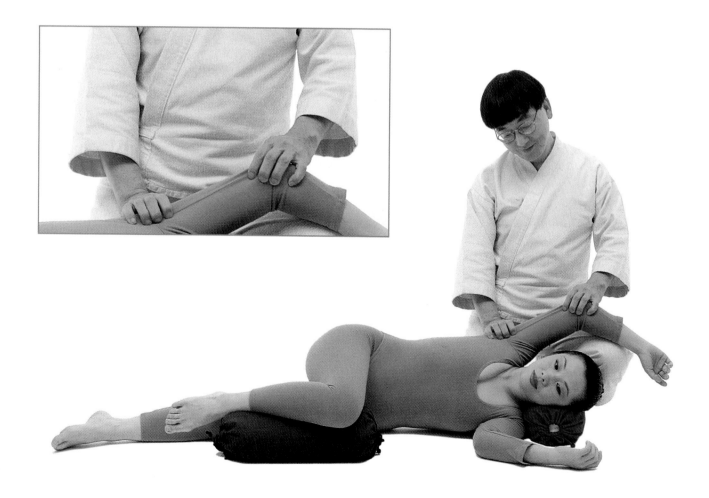

WORKING THE BACK AND LEGS

WORKING THE BACK

With the thumb and fingers

As you finish rotating the receiver's arm, turn your body so that you are once again parallel to her and facing her head; keep your left leg raised.

Next, slide your right hand under her right arm and up, to grasp the inside of her shoulder. Your left hand remains in place, with the fingers on the top of the shoulder and the thumb pressing into the area between the shoulder blade and the spine, around Bladder meridian tsubos #12 and #13 (see the meridian charts, page 4).

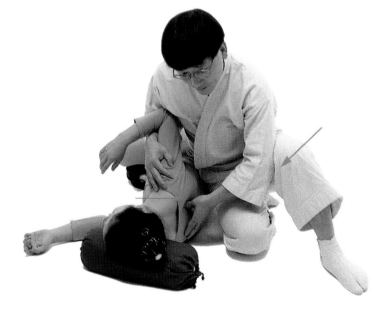

Bring her right shoulder toward you as you press with your thumb. If you want to penetrate more deeply, bring your left elbow against the inside of your left knee and then push forward with your knee. If the receiver feels pain from the pressure, squeeze her shoulder with your right hand.

If your thumb becomes tired, or if you want to give a different feeling, you may use four fingers instead of your thumb. Bring her shoulder toward you as your fingers first slip under the blade, then scoop forward.

Work down the meridian slowly, to tsubo #28 in the middle of the buttock. Press when she is breathing out; release when she is breathing in.

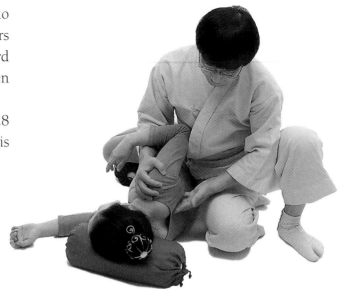

With the elbow

To slow the pace of a session (and to give yourself a chance to rest a little), you may want to use your elbow on the Bladder meridian (see "Elbow Technique," pages 60–61). I tend to use this technique when the receiver is big and there is more surface area on the back.

Remain parallel to the receiver's body (as you are when you use your thumb or fingers) but lower your left leg and extend it out to the side, away from the receiver. This lowers your center of gravity and helps you keep your balance while you use your elbow.

Your left (mother) hand remains across her right shoulder with your thumb in the area of Bladder #12 or #13, between the top of the shoulder blade and the spine. Apply the part of your

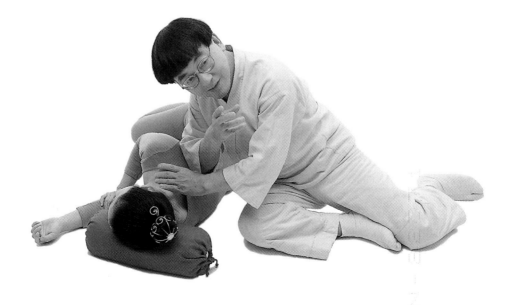

right forearm that is just below the elbow, parallel first, to the meridian in the area around tsubo #14 or #15 (your arm should be relaxed and open to about a 90-degree angle).

Lean toward her from your hara. If she can tolerate more pressure, slowly raise your forearm (to sharpen your elbow) and move your left leg further back (to maintain cross-patterning). Continue down the meridian to the middle of the buttock, around tsubo #27 or #28.

Note: Always apply your forearm parallel to the meridian, to prevent your sharpened elbow from slipping and hitting the spine, which could be very painful for the receiver. And be sure to keep the receiver from falling forward by pulling her toward you with your mother hand.

With palms

In order to work on the Bladder meridian with your palms when the receiver is on her side, you need to assume a crawling position, to distribute your body weight properly. To prevent her from falling forward as you apply your weight, first bring her right knee (still supported by a pillow) up closer to her hara. Second, be sure to support her firmly with your mother hand as described below.

Turn your body perpendicular to the receiver and get into a crawling position, with the thumb of your left (mother) hand between her shoulder blade and spine, in the area around Bladder #12 and #13, and your fingers across the top of her shoulder. Apply the palm of your right (messenger) hand between the shoulder blade and spine, a little further down the meridian, around the area of tsubos #14 and #15. Keep your spine straight and relaxed, and bring your hara toward her back. (Notice how far away I am from the receiver in the photograph.)

Palm down the meridian to the middle of the buttock, around tsubo #27 or #28. Make sure your left (messenger) knee moves as your right hand moves. For deeper penetration, you can use your thumb after you use your palm one or two times.

WORKING THE RIB CAGE AND HIPS

Remain parallel to the receiver, with your right knee down and your left knee raised. With your left hand, grasp the side of her rib cage about halfway down. Your fingers should be on her back and your thumb in the direction of her chest, at about Gall Bladder meridian tsubo #24 (see the meridian charts, page 6). Place your right hand just below your left hand (or with your left thumb overlapping your right forefinger), holding her rib cage in the same way but with fingers and thumb reversed. This hand position is called *tiger mouth.*

Lean in toward your hands and hold. Next, move your right hand down the meridian to the middle of the hip (around tsubo #30), leaning into the major tsubos along the way and moving your left leg back as you go. When you reach the hip, your right hand becomes the mother hand and your left hand becomes the messenger hand— which now moves down the meridian in the same manner. Be sure to move your right knee as you move your left hand.

The "tiger mouth" technique can also be done by leaning and pressing with both hands at the same time, from the armpit to the hip. There is no distinction between mother and messenger hands, but you still move your left leg toward your right knee.

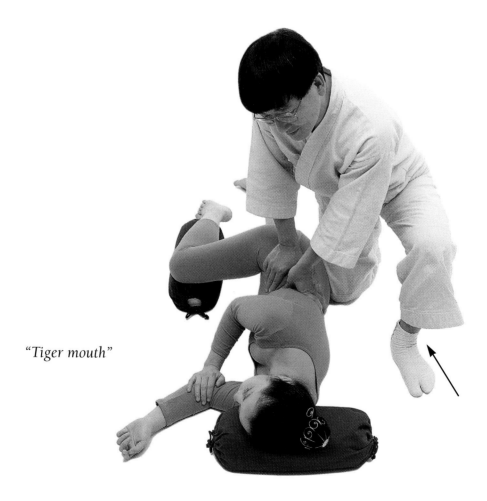

"Tiger mouth"

WORKING THE LEGS

Gall Bladder and Bladder meridians, upper leg

After you have worked the Gall Bladder meridian from the rib cage to the hip, keep both hands on the hip and lean into the receiver. While you are supporting your weight on your hands, raise your hips, bring your right leg over the receiver's body, and kneel down just in front of her knee. As you do so, raise your left leg. You will be astride the receiver's legs, facing her head.

Keep your left (mother) hand on the middle of her hip, around the area of Gall Bladder #30. With your right hand, work down the Gall Bladder meridian on the outside of the upper leg to the knee, using either your palm or your thumb. Do this two or three times, remembering to move your hara in a figure 8 and to move your messenger knee when you move your right hand.

Now work the Bladder meridian, which is toward the back of the thigh, in the same manner, from tsubo #36, just below the buttock, to tsubo #40, at the back of the kneecap (see the meridian charts, page 4). After you work it a few times with your right hand, keep that hand on the kneecap and work down it once with your left hand.

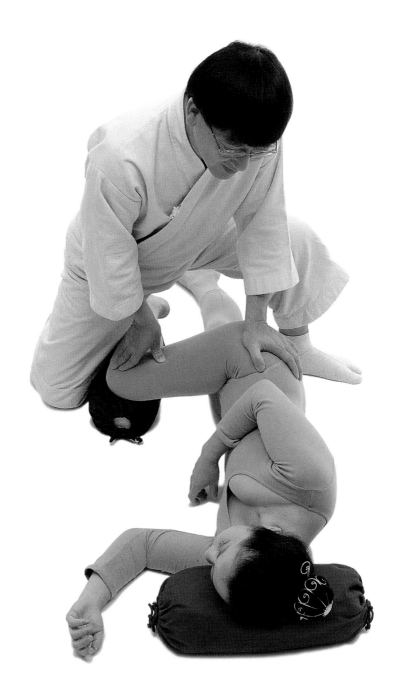

Gall Bladder and Bladder meridians, lower leg

With your left (mother) hand on the kneecap and your right (messenger) hand just beside it on the upper leg, lean toward the receiver and bring your right leg back beside your left (so that now both are on the same side of the receiver). You should now be facing the back of the receiver's lower leg.

Shift your left hand to the kneecap and, with your right hand, work down the Gall Bladder meridian on the outside of the lower leg (see the meridian charts, page 6) to just below the ankle, around tsubo #40. You may use either your palm or your thumb.

Next, repeat on the Bladder meridian, which runs down the back of the calf, then work toward the outside of the lower leg and down through the ankle to the little toe. You may have to turn the receiver's leg downward slightly to expose the meridian fully. After you have worked the meridian a few times with your right hand, keep that hand around Bladder tsubo #60 and work down the meridian once with your left hand.

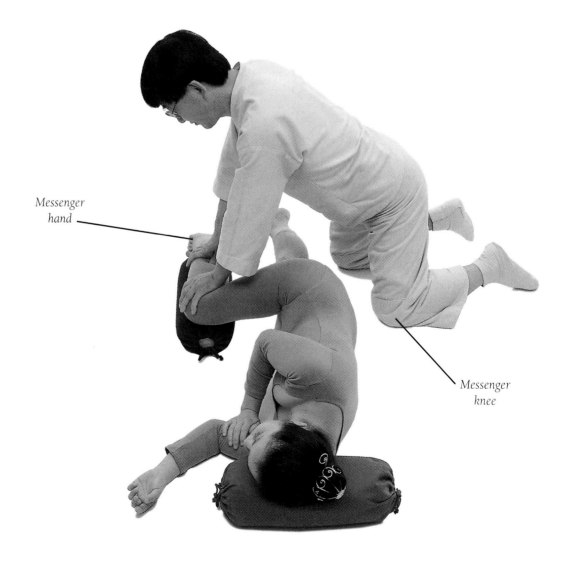

Messenger hand

Messenger knee

Spleen, Liver, and Kidney meridians, lower left leg

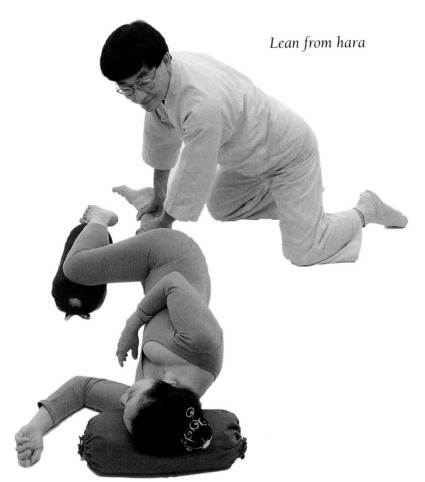

Lean from hara

After working the Gall Bladder and Bladder meridians in the right lower leg, release your hands and crawl sideways to your right so that you are facing the middle of the lower left leg. Hold the receiver's ankle with your right hand and put your left hand beside it. Now, you are in position to work the Spleen, Liver, and Kidney meridians—all yin meridians that run from the foot up—on the left leg (see the meridian charts, pages 3, 5, and 6).

Using your left hand as the messenger hand, work up the Spleen meridian (near the shinbone) to the knee two or three times with your palm. Next, do the same on the Liver meridian (along the center calf) and the Kidney meridian (along the outer calf). Use your thumb on these meridians only with extreme caution; the inside of the leg (both upper and lower) is very tender.

Spleen, Liver, and Kidney meridians, upper left leg

Crawl sideways to your left, so that you are about in the middle of the receiver's upper leg. Now, your right hand becomes the mother hand at her kneecap, and your left hand (as messenger hand) moves up the meridians, one after the other, from the kneecap to the top of the thigh. Then place your left hand (which now becomes the mother hand) on her sacrum and palm up the meridians once with your right (messenger) hand.

You are now ready to begin the stretching technique on the next page, or to make a transition to another part of the body, or to return to gasho if you have finished the session.

STRETCHING THE BODY

And working the Bladder meridian on the back

This technique looks difficult but is actually very easy, especially when the receiver has a big frame and is flexible. Because it stretches the entire body, it is a good technique to use at the end of each side.

Position yourself in a squat at the receiver's waistline. (If you cannot squat with both knees up, you can place the left knee on the floor or put a pillow under both knees.) Slide your right palm under her right kneecap and raise her leg toward you, so that it comes to rest on your right forearm. Slide your left hand under the outside of her right elbow, and extend her arm back along your left side.

Bring your right knee into her upper right thigh, in the area of Bladder meridian tsubo #37, and your left knee into

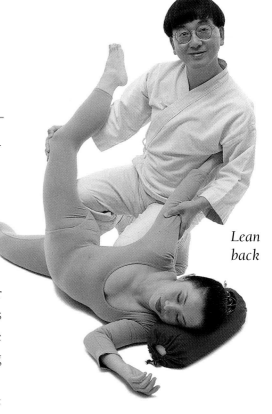

Lean back

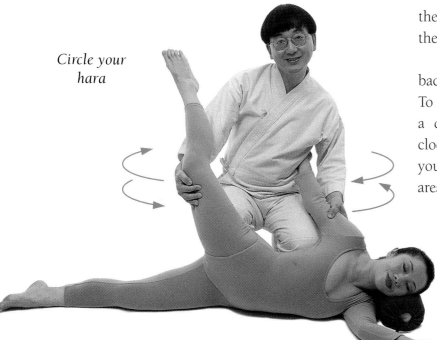

Circle your hara

the area between the shoulder blade and the spine, around tsubos #14 and #15.

Keeping your spine straight, lean back in order to stretch her arm and leg. To stretch even more, move your hara in a circle, either clockwise or counterclockwise. Next, lean forward, release your left knee, and move it down to the area of tsubos #18 and #19 on the Bladder meridian (see the meridian charts, page 4). Lean back again, to stretch the arm and leg.

Continue down the meridian until you reach her hip. Repeat several times.

And working the Stomach meridian on the upper leg

After working the Bladder meridian, keep your knees on her hip and upper leg, and release your left hand from her arm. Now, place your left hand at the top center of her right leg, around Stomach meridian tsubo #30, and work down the meridian to her kneecap with your fingers. At each major tsubo, lean back to stretch the leg; then lean forward, release, and move your fingers to the next tsubo. You will be gently squeezing as you pull against the Stomach meridian.

When you have finished working the meridian, return her arm and leg to their original positions (see page 143).

Now you are ready to turn her over in order to work on her left side (see transition on page 176). Follow the directions in this section, switching hands and knees.

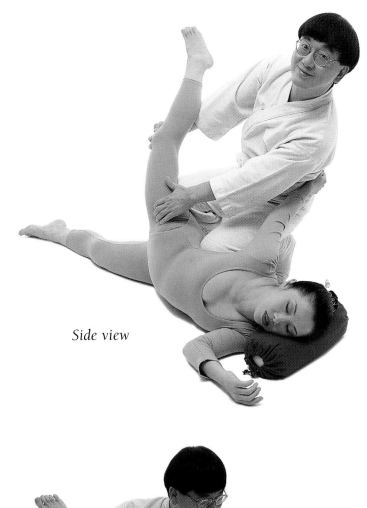

Side view

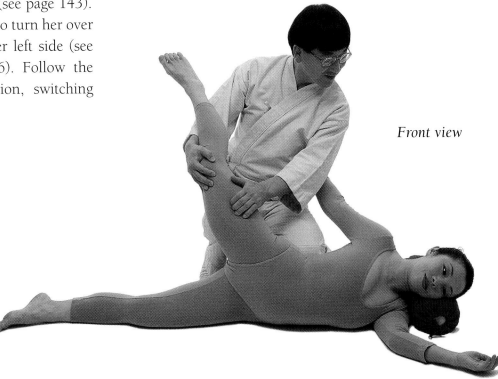

Front view

5

MOVING IN

TONUS . . .

THE SIT-UP

POSITION

One of the many advantages of Ohashiatsu is its convenience: You can practice the techniques almost anywhere because you don't need special equipment and the receiver does not need to remove his or her clothes. The sit-up position is especially practical: You can use the following sit-up techniques almost anytime and anywhere—just five or ten minutes of treatment can be beneficial, and you can do most of the techniques while the receiver is sitting in a chair.

Like the side position, the sit-up position may also be especially comfortable for those who are receiving Ohashiatsu for the first time. People don't usually mind being touched on their arms, shoulders, and back, but the front of the body and the legs are considered more personal; a receiver may be hesitant about being touched there until he trusts the giver.

The sitting position confines the giver's movements to an even smaller area than does the side position, but all the basic principles of Ohashiatsu still apply. When you work on a receiver in the sit-up position, the principle of support is extremely important (see "Supporting," pages 21–26). You want to keep the receiver from falling forward as you apply pressure, without keeping such a tense hold that you limit your own flexibility. This requires the establishment of mutual support—the more you lean toward the receiver, the more you pull him or her toward you. Cross-patterning still applies, too—although more subtly than with the other positions. When your mother hand supports the shoulder, your mother knee supports the back. When your messenger hand moves along a meridian, your messenger knee moves as well (although your leg remains in place). And, of course, you should always remember to stay in tonus and keep your spine straight.

You will notice that I have included techniques for the Large Intestine, Triple Heater, and Small Intestine meridians, yang meridians that run down the outside and back of the arm. I have chosen to present them here, but they may also be worked on when the receiver is in the side position.

Most of the techniques in this section can be applied to both sides of the body. In the interest of brevity, I have demonstrated them on only the left side. You can begin on either side, and after you have finished a sequence on one side of the receiver, simply slide to the other side (keeping one hand on the body) and repeat the techniques, switching your hand and leg positions.

Preparation

Make sure the receiver is seated comfortably. If you are working on the floor, I find that a cross-legged position (with the forearms resting, palms up, on the thighs and the spine straight but relaxed) is usually the best for the receiver. However, she can also leave her legs outstretched; she can even be seated in a chair.

Before you begin, perform gashyo, or just close your eyes for a minute or two, to focus yourself. Rub down your hands, if necessary.

STRETCHING THE SHOULDERS AND ARMS

Sequence

- ◆ Warming up the shoulders

    With the palms

    With the elbows

- ◆ Stretching the arms and spine

    Overhead stretch

    "Chicken-wing" stretch

- ◆ Working the arms

    Arm rotation

    Working the Lung
    meridian (yin)

Working the Large
Intestine meridian (yang)

Working the Heart
Constrictor meridian (yin)

Working the Triple Heater
meridian (yang)

Working the Heart
meridian (yin)

Working the Small
Intestine meridian (yang)

Working the other arm

WARMING UP THE SHOULDERS

With the palms

Stand centered behind the receiver and apply both hands on her shoulders, near the base of her neck, in the area of Gall Bladder meridian tsubo #21 (see the meridian charts, page 6). Apply your right knee to the *left* side of her back, in the area between the spine and the left shoulder blade, around Bladder meridian tsubos #15 and #16.

When she is breathing out, lean

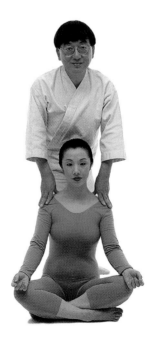

Front view

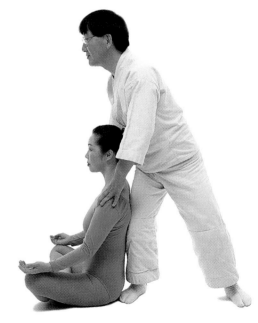

Side view

toward her from your hara and, simultaneously, pull her back toward you; you should be supporting each other. Lean and release about three times, moving your palms out to the edge of her shoulders.

After using your palms, you may repeat with your thumb—for deeper penetration. Be careful not to press suddenly; communicate verbally with the receiver about how much pressure she can tolerate.

If the receiver is small, you may kneel behind her with your left knee raised out to the side and your right leg supporting her back. If you have to bend your elbows in this position, be careful to continue to use your body weight and not press with your arm muscles alone.

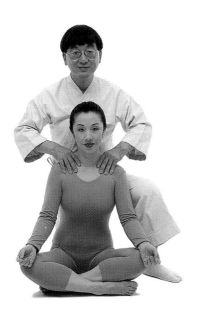

Front view

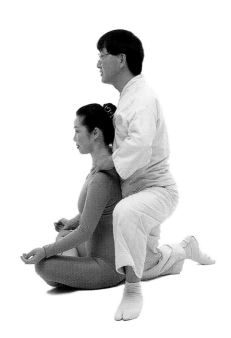

Side view

⊘ DON'T! ─────────────────────────

I am standing too far away from the receiver and can't lean with my full body weight. My back is rounded and I'm relying only on muscle power in my arms and fingers. To practice this technique correctly, I should always keep my spine and legs in a straight line, and my arms and the receiver's spine in a straight line.

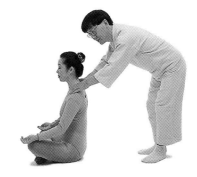

With the elbows

For even deeper penetration, you can also use your elbows on the shoulders.

Kneel behind the receiver with either your hara or your right leg supporting her back and your left leg raised. Place the lower part of your forearms (just above the elbows) in the area of Gall Bladder tsubo #21, near the base of the neck on both shoulders. Lean in from your hara and hold for a few seconds. Then lean back, release, and move your forearms to the next major tsubo. Continue outward along the shoulders. Then return to the base of the neck and repeat. If you want more pressure at any point, raise your forearms slowly, so that the pressure shifts toward your elbows (which I call sharpening the elbow).

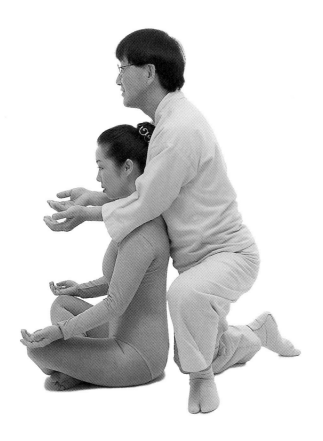

Using forearms

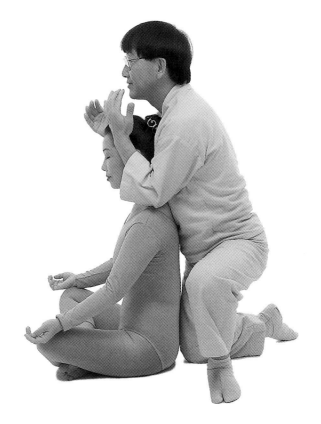

Sharpening the elbow

STRETCHING THE ARMS AND SPINE

Overhead stretch

This stretch transition is good for correcting bad posture, alleviating tension in the back, and treating breathing difficulties.

From a standing position, with the side of your right leg supporting the receiver's back to the left of her spine, slide your hands off the receiver's shoulders and down her upper arms. Grasp her elbows and bring the arms over her head as you slide your hands to her wrists. Lean back to stretch her arms. Push forward with your right leg to stretch more. Repeat several times.

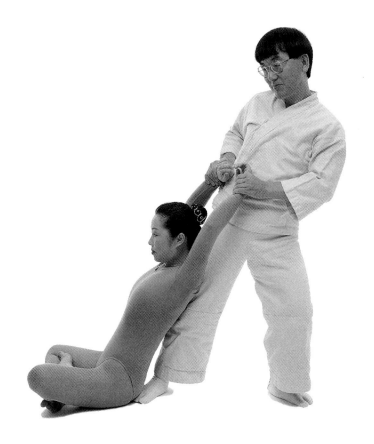

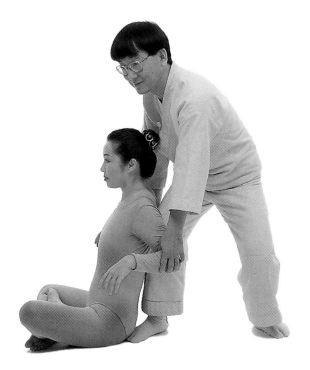

"Chicken-wing" stretch

Slide your hands to her elbows and lower her arms to a "chicken-wing" position. Next, bring her elbows back toward you, hold two or three seconds, then extend them in front of her in a swooping motion. Bring the arms into the chicken-wing position again and repeat the entire sequence. Support her back with the side of your right leg.

After you have done this technique a few times, move behind her left side and lower her arms to begin work on her left arm.

WORKING THE ARMS

Here, you will be working on both yin and yang meridians, alternating between the two, to provide balance. You will work only with your fingers or your thumb; the area is too small for the palm.

Arm rotation

This rotation enables you to get a sense of the arm's flexibility as you make the transition from one meridian to the next when you work on the arm. If you can rotate it with little or no resistance, the receiver can probably tolerate a fairly high amount of stretching.

Kneel down on your right knee so that it supports her left hip. Raise your left leg out to the side. Put your right (mother) hand on her left shoulder, with your thumb in the area between the shoulder blade and the spine. With your left hand hold her left arm just below the elbow and extend it out in front of her.

Now, rotate her arm in as wide a circle as possible, both clockwise and counterclockwise, two or three times. Keep her body stabilized with your mother hand, squeezing her shoulder and pressing with your thumb.

This arm rotation is an important transition technique to use when you move from one meridian to another. It is an opportunity for you to place your body in the right position for the next meridian, thereby making a smooth transition. I usually rotate the arm three times, but you can decide.

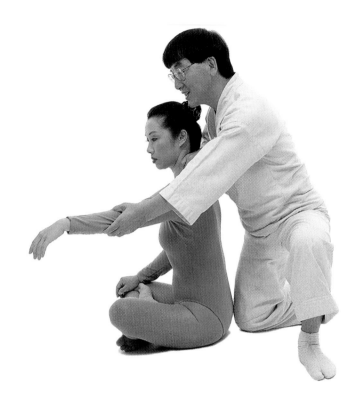

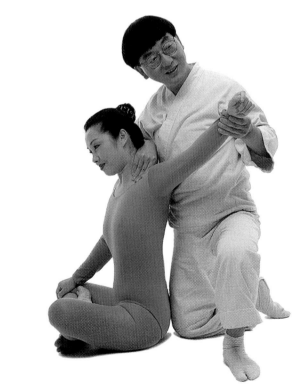

Working the Lung meridian (yin)

As you finish rotating the receiver's arm, your right fingers should grasp Lung tsubo #1, in the hollow area just below the outer end of her collarbone.

With your left hand, bring her left arm back to rest on your left knee. Now, place your left hand beside your right one.

When she breathes out, lean back and, pulling her arm toward you, squeeze with both hands. (Remember: Feeling the same amount of pressure from both hands is more comfortable for the receiver. It also creates an echo effect; that is, a sensation along the entire meridian.)

Hold the squeeze for a few seconds, then release when she is breathing in and move your left fingers up to the next major tsubo. Repeat up the meridian to Lung tsubo #9, just below the base of her thumb.

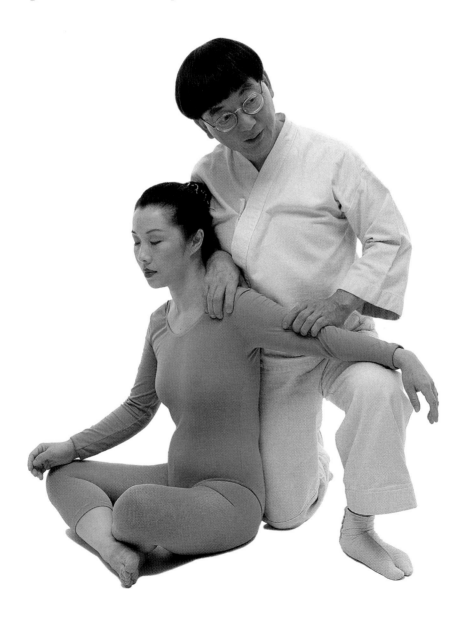

Working the Large Intestine meridian (yang)

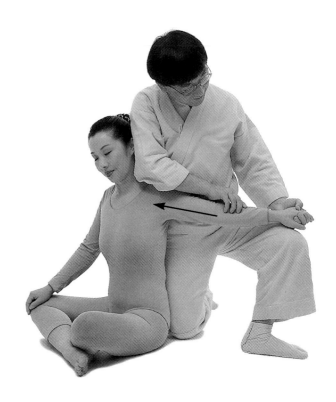

Rotate the receiver's arm again, and as you finish, bring her arm back, palm down, and rest it on your left knee. Continue to support her back with your right leg. Hold her hand with your left thumb on top and your fingers underneath, their tips holding the area along the inside of her index finger, at Large Intestine meridian tsubo #4 (see the meridian charts, page 2). Move your right hand (now the messenger hand) to her wrist, just beside your left (mother) hand. Work down the meridian (which runs along the outside edge of the arm) with your right hand to the area of Large Intestine #15, just below the front edge of her shoulder. Along the way, lean back and squeeze with both hands at the major tsubos. To stretch more at any point, push her forward with your right leg as you lean back. Work slowly.

Working the Heart Constrictor meridian (yin)

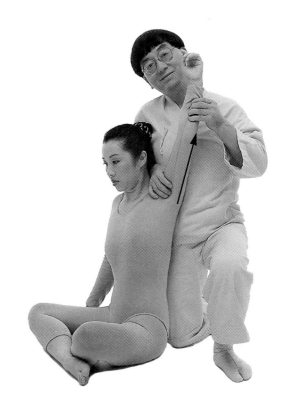

Rotate the receiver's arm again, and as you finish, place her raised arm, palm outward, on your chest for support. Shift the fingers of your right hand to Heart Constrictor tsubo #2, at the outer edge of the armpit, and bring your left hand (now the messenger hand) beside it.

When she breathes out, squeeze both hands and lean back to stretch her arm. (If you want to stretch her arm more at any point, you can move your left leg back and push forward with your right leg.)

Work up the meridian in this way along the middle of her inner arm to the center of her wrist, the area of Heart Constrictor #7 (see the meridian charts, page 5).

Working the Triple Heater meridian (yang)

Rotate the receiver's arm, and as you finish, lower your left knee to the floor and bring her arm back toward you with her palm facing inward, to expose the Triple Heater meridian, which runs along the back of the arm (see the meridian charts, page 5).

Hold her hand from underneath, with your left fingers pressing in between the bones just below her fourth and fifth fingers, in the area of Triple Heater tsubo #3. Put your right hand beside your left hand. Your right knee still supports her hip.

When she breathes out, squeeze both hands, lean back, and pull her arm toward you. Work down the meridian with your right hand, to the top center of the upper arm just below the tip of the shoulder, in the area of Triple Heater #14. Remember to push forward with your right knee if you want to stretch the arm more.

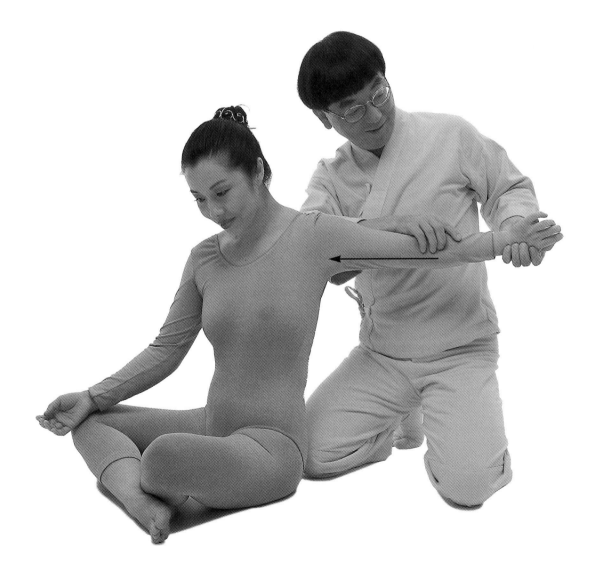

Working the Heart meridian (yin)

Rotate the receiver's arm, then raise your left knee and bring her upper arm to rest on your chest, with her forearm bent down behind her head. Shift your right fingers to hold Heart tsubo #1, in the front of her armpit (see the meridian charts, page 3). Place your left hand beside your right hand.

   When she breathes out, squeeze both hands and lean back to the right side. When she breathes in, release the pressure and move your left hand to the next major tsubo. Work up the meridian in this manner along the innermost edge of the arm to the tip of her little finger, Heart #9.

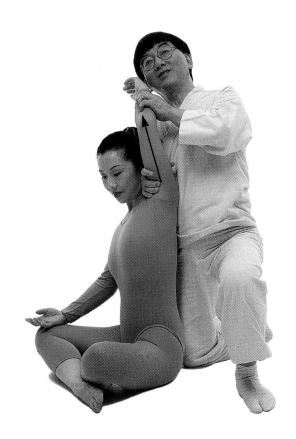

Working the Small Intestine meridian (yang)

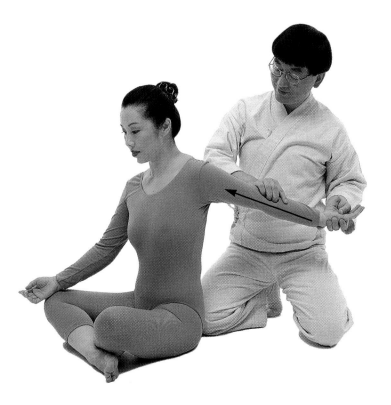

Rotate the receiver's arm again. Next, bring your left knee back down, and bring her arm back toward you, fully extended and palm up, to expose the Small Intestine meridian, which runs along the back of the arm (see the meridian charts, page 3). With the fingers of your left hand (now the mother hand), hold her hand in the area just below the knuckle of the little finger, around Small Intestine tsubo #3. Place your right hand beside your left hand.

   When she is breathing out, squeeze with both hands and lean back to stretch her arm. When she is breathing in, release and move your right hand to the next major tsubo. Proceed down the meridian to the back of her shoulder, the area of Small Intestine #15 (see meridian charts, page 3).

From one arm to the other

After working the meridians in the receiver's left arm, rotate that arm again. Then stand and stretch both arms over her head and move to her right side. Kneel down on your left knee so that it is supporting her right hip, and raise your right knee out to the side. Now, rotate her right arm and repeat the techniques given on pages 152–156, switching your hands and knees accordingly.

After you have finished working on the right arm, rotate that arm again a few times, lower your right knee, and move your torso so that you are kneeling directly behind the receiver. Place your hands on her shoulders and squeeze them a couple of times. Now you are ready to begin the head rotation.

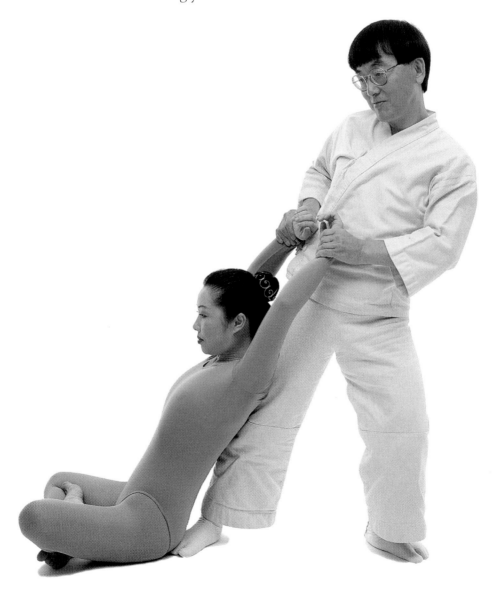

Sequence

HANDS ON THE HEAD

- ◆ Head rotation, squeezing the temples
- ◆ Thumb technique while grasping
- ◆ Holding the forehead
- ◆ Scooping technique
- ◆ Fingers on the forehead

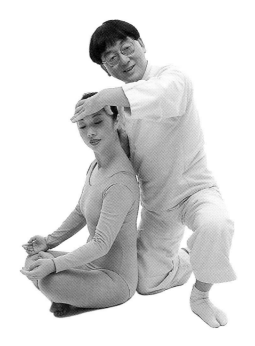

Head rotation, squeezing the temples

I begin work on the neck, head, and face with a head rotation, which I also repeat after each technique. (The rotation is also good for relieving headache, nausea, and tension.)

Slowly raise your left leg, and move your left hand to her forehead: Apply the thumb of your left hand to the receiver's left temple; apply the middle finger of your left hand to her right temple, at Gall Bladder tsubo #1 on each side (see the meridian charts, page 6). Apply the thumb and middle finger of your right hand to Gall Bladder #20, at the base of her skull on each side of her head.

When she breathes out, squeeze both hands gently but firmly while you rotate her head in as wide a circle as her flexibility allows. Be sure to move very slowly. Breathe with her and move your hara as you rotate her head. Rotate clockwise and counterclockwise, two or three times in each direction.

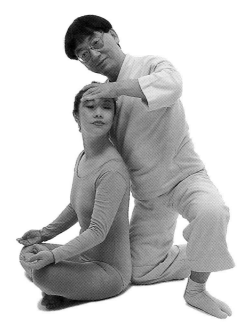

Thumb technique while grasping

This technique is good for relieving headache.

Place your thumbs on both sides of the receiver's head at Gall Bladder tsubo #20. Spread the fingers of both hands and grasp her head just above the ears, in the area of her temples. (Your palms should be arched over her ears.)

When she breathes out, bring her head toward you as you lean back, and at the same time press upward with your thumbs. If she feels pain, release the pressure from your thumbs and fingers and rotate her head two or three times gently in each direction; then, try to apply pressure with your thumbs again.

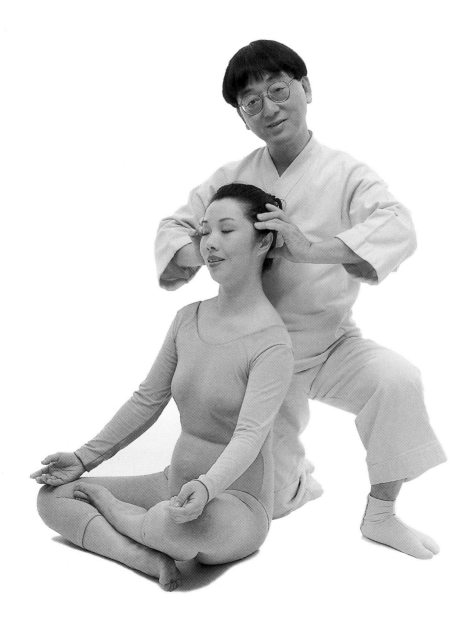

Holding the forehead

After leaning into Gall Bladder tsubo #20 with your thumbs, rotate her head again. As you rotate, place your left thumb on Governing Vessel meridian tsubo #16, the groove in the center of the base of her cranium (at the top of the spine). Bring back her head toward your left thumb when she is breathing out, then squeeze with both hands for two to three seconds, as these photographs illustrate.

If she wants stronger and deeper pres-

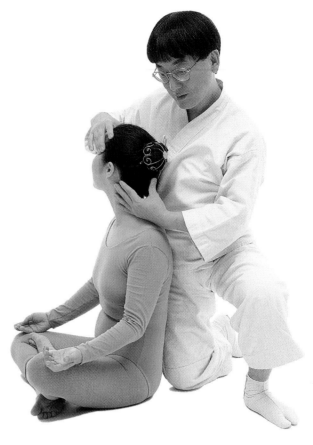

sure, rest your left elbow on your left knee, in order to support your arm; your right fingers hold both temples. When she breathes out, bring her body back toward you. If she can tolerate even more pressure, lift your left heel, which will cause your thumb to go deeper. Then release the pressure and rotate her head one or two times. Apply pressure again, and rotate again. If the receiver is tense, continue to rotate her head until she surrenders to the movement. (If her neck remains tense, discontinue the rotation and go to another technique.) Sometimes during this procedure I vibrate my hands.

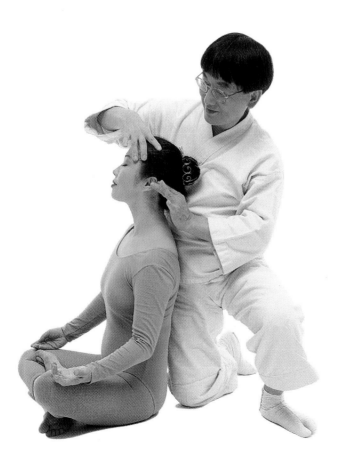

Fingers on the forehead

Use this for the relief of headache and insomnia.

Raise your left leg and support the receiver's back with your right leg. Apply four fingers of each hand just under her eyebrows, and pull upward when she breathes out. When she breathes in, release your fingers and move them a little bit further up her forehead; then, pull upward again. Repeat at several places until you reach her hairline.

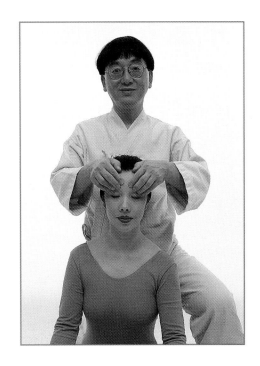

Scooping technique

This technique helps relieve nasal and sinus congestion.

Support the receiver's head against your chest. Apply your middle finger of each hand under each cheekbone and *scoop* her face up toward you; her head will tilt back slightly. Next apply three fingers and scoop again.

If the receiver's face is oily, do only one cheekbone at a time. Place your other palm over her eye to protect it, in case your fingers slip.

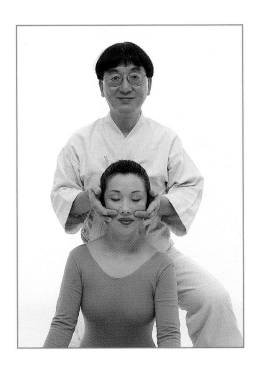

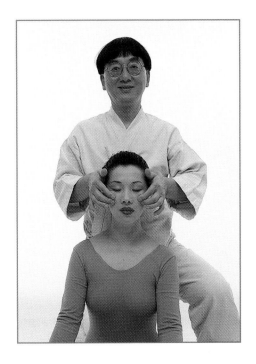

LOOSENING THE SHOULDERS AND BACK

Sequence

◆ Shoulders with one elbow

◆ Neck and shoulder squeeze

◆ Working the Back

  With one palm

  With one elbow

  With one thumb

  With two thumbs

  Palm down spine

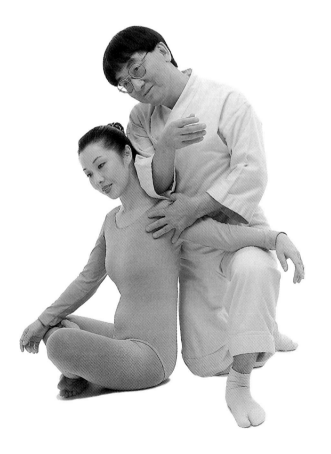

Shoulders with one elbow

After you have finished working on the head and face, move back to the left side of the receiver's body. Kneel down on your right knee, raise your left knee out to the side, and rotate her left arm. Bring her left arm back to rest on your left knee, palm down. Place your right arm—the forearm, just above the elbow—on her left shoulder near her neck, in the area of Gall Bladder tsubo #21 (see the meridian charts, page 6). With your left hand hold the front edge of her shoulder.

When she breathes in, pull her body toward you by leaning back from your hara. (When I say pull, I don't mean jerk; the movement should be firm but smooth.) When she breathes out, slowly shift your body weight to your elbow by leaning toward her. If she seems to be falling forward, pull her closer toward you. Your right leg can be against the receiver's body to support her if she needs it.

If she wants more pressure, sharpen your elbow as described on page 61.

ELBOW TECHNIQUE IN THE SIT-UP POSITION

When you use your elbow in the sit-up position, you must make sure that the pressure does not cause the receiver to fall forward. Keep her spine straight and support it with your leg. Lean toward her first, then pull her toward you—so that you are supporting each other (see "Supporting," pages 21–26).

Don't use the tip of your elbow at first; use the part of your forearm that is near the elbow, and ask her if she feels uncomfortable. If she says she can tolerate more pressure, you may raise your forearm, to shift your weight onto the elbow itself. On each tsubo, begin in the softer position (forearm open and relaxed), then sharpen the elbow to achieve deeper penetration.

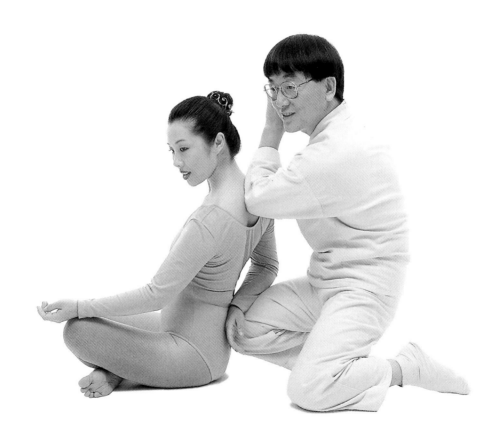

Neck and shoulder squeeze

Rest the receiver's left arm on your left leg, and hold the front edge of her left shoulder with your left hand. Put your right thumb on the bottom of her skull, just behind her left ear (Gall Bladder #20), with your right fingers around the back of her neck.

When she breathes out, squeeze both hands and lean in with your right hand and pull in the opposite direction with your left, stretching the neck and shoulder area on the Gall Bladder meridian. Be sure to support her with your left hand. Repeat two or three times.

Now, rotate her left arm and move away from the receiver's body into a squat, with your right knee on the floor and your left knee up. This puts you into a position to work on her back.

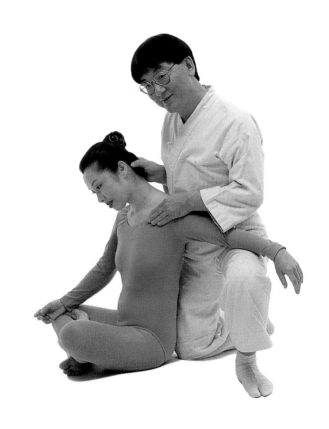

WORKING THE BACK

With one palm

Keep the receiver's back straight and hold the edge of her left shoulder with your left hand. Put your right hand between her spine and her shoulder blade on the left side of her back, in the area of Bladder tsubos #13, #14, and #15 (see the meridian charts, page 4).

When she breathes out, lean into the meridian and pull her shoulder back. Now, slide your right palm down the meridian to her lower back, around tsubo #23. Repeat a couple of times.

For deeper penetration, you may also do this technique with your thumb, moving it down the meridian from tsubo to tsubo, rather than sliding.

With one elbow

Keep your left leg raised.

Raise your right knee and support her left hip. With your left hand, bring the receiver's left arm behind her back and rest it at the wrist against your right knee. This position helps you to keep her balanced as you work.

Next, return your left hand to her left shoulder and put your right forearm (near your elbow) between her left shoulder blade and her spine.

Lean toward her and pull her shoulder back toward you. If she wants deeper penetration, slowly sharpen your elbow by bending your forearm. Hold for three to five seconds. If she can tolerate even more, first pull her shoulder back further, then lean toward her again. Continue down the meridian to the lower back, around the area of Bladder #23.

Here, once more, the principle of supporting and being supported applies: Let her body beckon to your elbow.

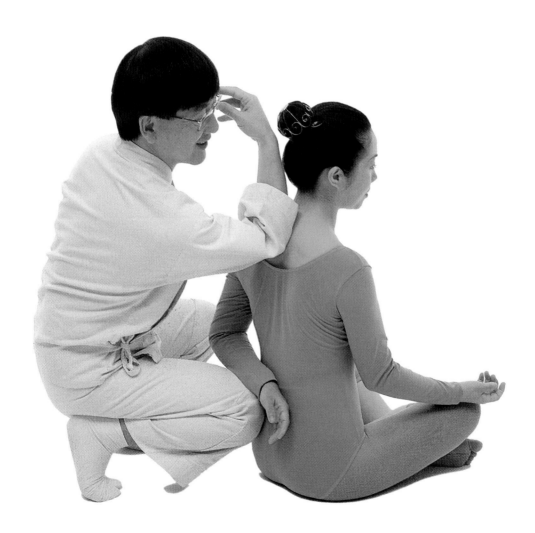

With one thumb

For the deepest penetration, repeat the previous technique with your thumb. You may bring the receiver's left arm back to rest on your right knee, to help maintain her balance. Pull back your hara in a partial circle toward your right as you stretch.

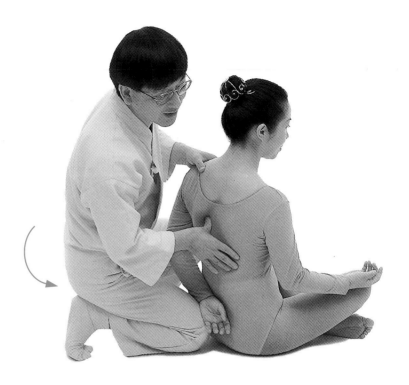

Palm down spine

After you have finished a sequence of techniques on the back, slide your right palm down the receiver's spine, the Governing Vessel meridian (see the meridian charts, page 7), to the lower back a couple of times, to relax the receiver.

You may then rotate both arms simultaneously by grasping them at the elbow. Then, move to the right side of the receiver, switch hand and knee positions, and repeat the techniques described in this section.

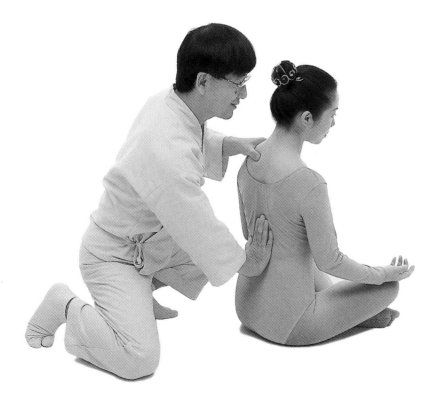

With two thumbs

At the very end of a session in the sit-up position, I center myself again behind the receiver and use this technique with two thumbs. Place four fingers of each hand across the top of the receiver's shoulders and your thumbs in the area of Bladder #12 on both sides of her spine. Lean toward your thumbs and bring her shoulders back toward you. Release the pressure, move your thumbs down to the next major tsubo (keeping your fingers in place), and lean again. Continue down the meridian as far as you can without releasing your fingers, to the area of tsubos #15 and #16.

Now, place your hands on her shoulders, close your eyes, and synchronize your breathing with hers to end the session.

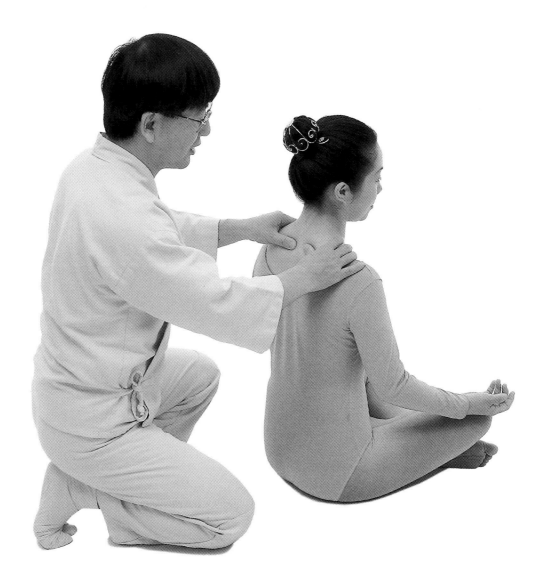

CHAIR TECHNIQUES

Today, there is a phenomenon called "seated massage" which has become popular with busy office workers who may not have time to travel to another location for a session. Most of the Ohashiatsu techniques in this section can be used on-site, with the receiver sitting in a chair; you will probably have to stand (rather than kneel) for most of them. For some of the techniques, you will need to have the receiver sit sideways, to give you access to certain areas of the back. Otherwise, just be sure to follow the basic principles of Ohashiatsu—Pull, don't press; use two hands; be natural; be continuous—in order to maximize the benefits for you and for the receiver.

PART III

Designing Your Own Session

———◆———

*The way we deal with energy is
the way we deal with life.*

6

THE ART

OF

TRANSITION

Once you have practiced working on a receiver in each of the Ohashiatsu positions, and you feel comfortable making transitions from one technique to another and applying sequences of techniques to different parts of the body, you will be ready to learn how to move the receiver from one position to another, so that you can use several positions in a single session.

Part II showed how to change the receiver from face-up to face-down, then from face-down to face-up. You can, in fact, change the receiver from any one of the basic positions to any other. Learning to make such changes gives you greater flexibility in designing an Ohashiatsu session suitable for your own size and ability, the receiver's condition, and the amount of time you have available.

Over the past 25 years, I have developed many different techniques for changing the receiver's position, and I have tried many different sequences of positions. They cannot all be described in this chapter, but you will find one example for each of the possible transitions. If you study them, you will discover how to adapt them to your own and the receiver's needs.

It is most important to prepare for these changes: Each technique in a session should get you into position for the next technique, and all the techniques in one position should lead toward making a transition into another position. I call this *micro change leading to macro change*. As you

work on a yang meridian in the leg, for instance, you move little by little (micro change with your hands and knees) down the receiver's body, so that you will be ready to work on a yin meridian (macro change from yang to yin), going up the body. Changing the receiver's position is a macro change, but in order for the change to be smooth and efficient, it should be preceded by carefully orchestrated smaller (micro) changes.

You may think I am making too much of the need for smooth transitions, but my experience has taught me that both the giver and the receiver benefit from them: The giver experiences less strain and fatigue; the receiver gains a sense of endless time and increased security. When you are good at making smooth transitions, the receiver may not even notice when he or she is being moved. (I have been able to change the position of sleeping clients without waking them up.) Well-executed transitions are among the things that Ohashiatsu is famous for. They are an important aspect of the principle of continuity.

You may use three or more positions for the receiver in any given session, if the receiver is receptive and you have the time. Again, the number and order of the techniques you use will be up to you. On page 182 I provide you with an index of the micro transitions already presented in Part II of this book. In Chapter 7, there are some sample sequences, to give you an idea of how different needs can determine various combinations.

MACRO TRANSITIONS:
CHANGING THE RECEIVER'S POSITION

From face-up . . .

. . . to face-down   (See pages 96–97.)

. . . to right-side-up

Take a kneeling position parallel to and about midway up the receiver's right side; place both hands on his hara. Have pillows ready to support his head and left knee. (If you are on the receiver's left side, reverse the instructions for your hand and leg positions.)

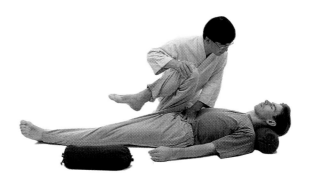

Slowly, slide your right hand down his right thigh, to the back of his knee. Lift his leg, move your hand around to hold his kneecap, and rotate his leg two or three times. Be sure to keep your left (mother) hand on his hara. After rotating, scoop your hand under his knee once more. Next, slide your left hand up the center of his chest (along the Conception Vessel meridian), over to his right shoulder, and down his right arm to his wrist. Now, move his right leg over to his left side, and rest his right knee on a pillow.

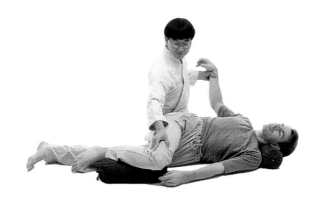

Bring your right hand up his thigh and along the side of his rib cage to hold the front of his right shoulder. With your right hand, drape his arm over your right forearm. Intertwine the fingers of your right and left hands over the top of his shoulders, then rotate his shoulder. (See the Side Position chapter on pages 128–145 for the techniques that follow this transition.)

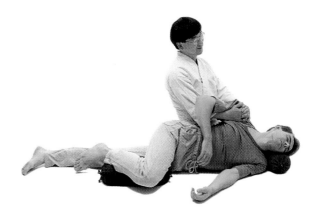

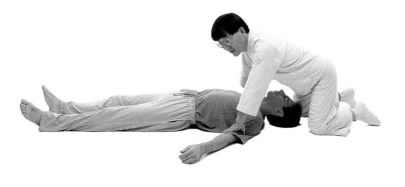

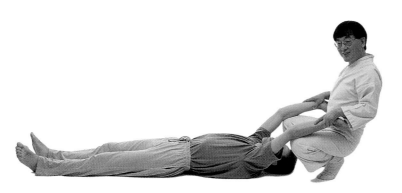

. . . to sit-up

From a kneeling position behind the receiver's head, put your right hand on his right shoulder and your left hand on his left shoulder. Slide both hands down his arms to his wrists, pick them up, and lean back to stretch them a couple of times. When you stretch his arms, your knees lift off the floor into a squat. Now, apply your knees to the back of his forearms and slowly stand and move to his side, bringing him with you into a sit-up position.

Immediately move behind him and support either side of his back with the side of your right leg. Stretch his arms toward the ceiling a couple of times, then bend them and bring them down against his sides, sliding your hands back from his wrists to his elbows. (See the Sit-Up Position chapter on pages 146–168 for the techniques that follow this transition.)

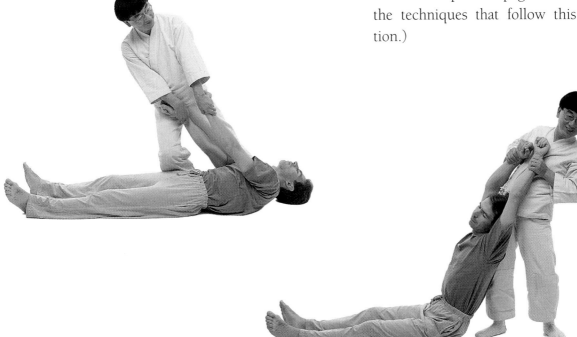

From face-down . . .

. . . to face-up   (See page 115.)

. . . to right-side-up

Take a kneeling position perpendicular to and about midway up the receiver's left side. Have a pillow in place to support his head at the end of the transition. Slide your left hand down the receiver's left arm, pick it up at the wrist, and stretch it out on the floor above and near his head.

Slide your right hand down the back of his right upper leg, grasp the back of his kneecap and slide the leg up toward his chest as far as it can comfortably go. Next, bring your left hand over to grasp the front of his right shoulder. Pull his shoulder and his right hip toward you so that he is now on his side.

Slide a pillow under his head. (Some receivers may also need a pillow under the bent knee.) Then with your right hand, drape his right arm over your forearm. Intertwine the fingers of your right and left hands over the top of his shoulder, and begin to rotate the shoulder. (See the Side Position chapter on pages 128–145 for the techniques that follow this transition.)

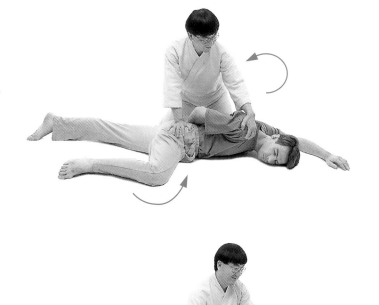

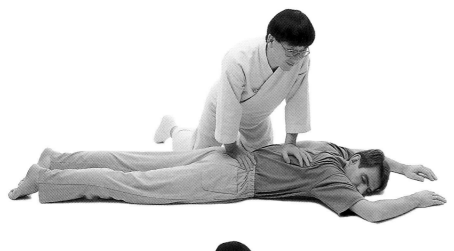

... to sit-up

Take a kneeling position perpendicular to and about midway up either side of the receiver. The receiver's arms should be above his head with palms down.

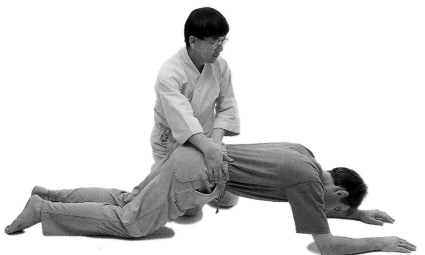

Grasp his hips with both hands and pull him back onto his heels. (The receiver may have to help.)

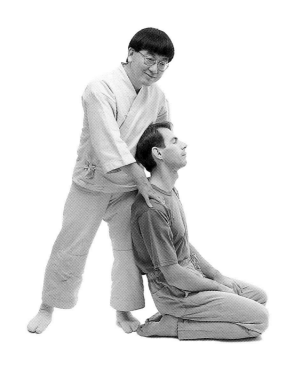

As you pull back, you stand up, and move behind him to support his back with your leg. (He can be in seiza, or rearrange his legs so that he is sitting cross-legged).

You are now in position to begin work on his shoulders. (See the Sit-Up Position chapter on pages 146–168 for the techniques that follow this transition.)

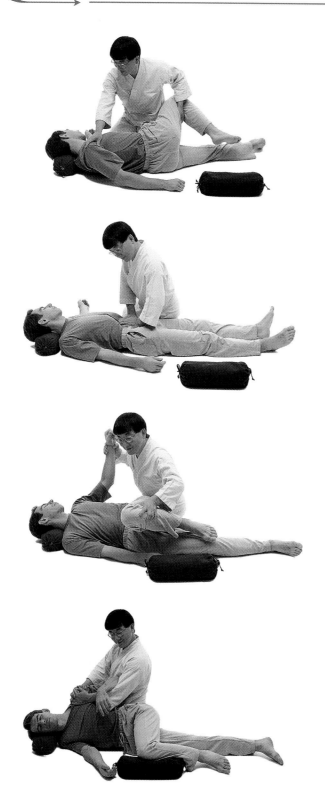

From side . . .

. . . to side

After you have finished working on the receiver's right side, place your right hand gently on his shoulder, move around his body in a squat-walk, and sit in seiza facing his hara. Slide your right hand under the outside of his right elbow (which is resting on his side), raise your hips, and lift his arm over and around his head and lower it to the floor behind him (his face will naturally turn up as you do this).

Next, loop your left hand under his right kneecap, bring it toward you and rotate his leg upward and outward. As you rotate, slide your right hand down the center of his chest (the Conception Vessel meridian) to his hara. Now, lower his right leg to the floor so that he is in a face-up position. Bring your left hand to his hara beside your right hand.

Next, slide your left hand down his left leg under the knee, pick it up, and rotate it. Meanwhile, slide your right hand from the hara up the Conception Vessel meridian to his left shoulder and down his arm to grasp his wrist or elbow. Holding his left wrist and knee, turn him onto his right side (left-side-up). Support his neck and left knee with pillows.

You are now ready to repeat the Side Position techniques of Chapter 4 (see pages 128–145) on the receiver's left side. Begin by raising your right leg, intertwining the fingers of both hands around his left shoulder, and rotating.

. . . to face-up

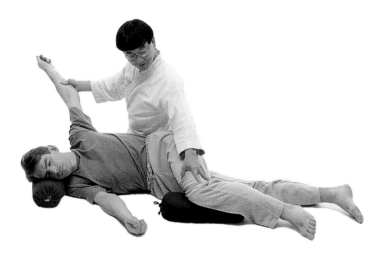

From a position about midway up the receiver's back.

When you finish working on the receiver's left side, rotate his left arm, and as you are rotating, lower that shoulder to the floor. Slide your left (messenger) hand from his shoulder, down along the side of his rib cage and the thigh of his left leg to his knee.

Scoop your hand under his knee and lift his leg toward you. (He will now be face-up.) Slide your left hand around to the front of his kneecap and rotate his leg. While you are rotating, slide your right hand down from his arm, along the center of his chest, to his hara. Straighten his left leg and lower it to the floor. (See pages 53–95 for the techniques that follow this transition.)

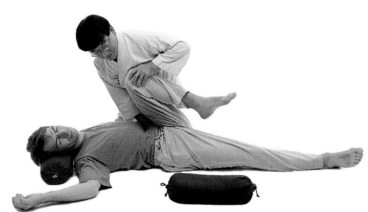

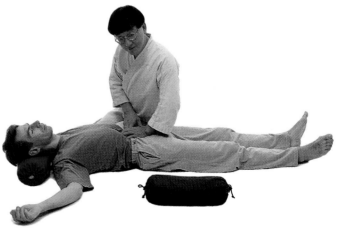

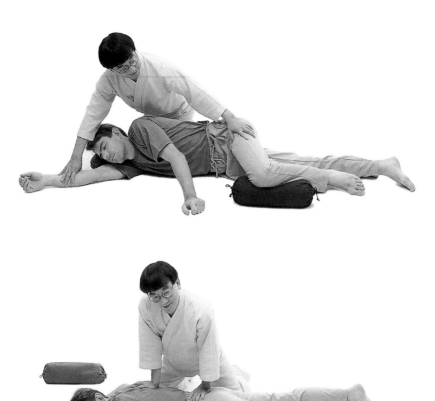

. . . to face-down

From a position parallel to and about midway up the back of the receiver, who is lying with his left side up.

With your right hand, bring the receiver's right arm up in front of his face, so that it is extended on the floor above his head. Next, move your right hand to his left shoulder and slide your left hand down his side, remove the pillow under his knee, and grasp his left kneecap. Your right hand remains on his left shoulder. Then, lean into him and roll him face-down with both hands. Remove the pillow that was supporting his head, and arrange his arms comfortably.

You will be in a crawling position, ready to work on his back (see page 96).

. . . to sit-up

From a position about midway up the back of the receiver, who is lying on either side.

Move the receiver into a face-up position, (see page 177) and then from face-up into sit-up (see page 173). Now you may do sit-up techniques (pages 146–168).

From sit-up . . .

. . . to face-up

From a squatting position behind the receiver.

Rotate both of his arms together a couple of times, then stand and stretch them up toward the ceiling, supporting his back with the side of your right leg.

Slowly, release your supporting leg, keep a firm grasp on his arms, and gradually move back to lower him onto the floor.

Now you may do neck (see pages 82–95) or face (see pages 119–127) techniques, or you may rotate the receiver's right arm in order to move down his right side to his hara to begin work on the legs (see pages 54–70).

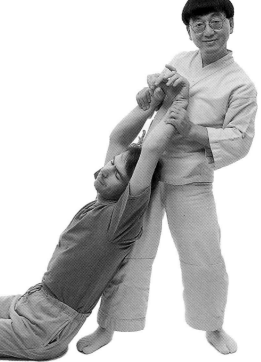

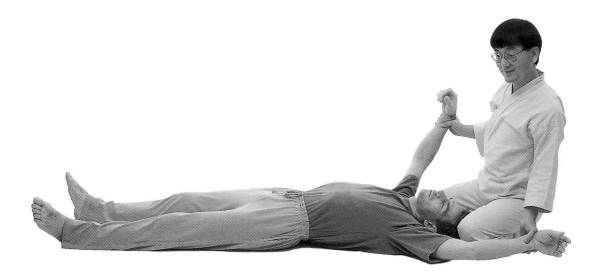

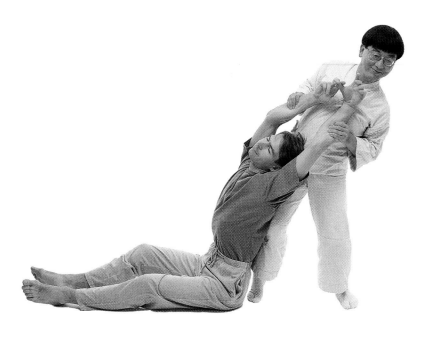

. . . to face-down

From a squatting position behind the receiver, rotate both of his arms.

Next, stand and stretch them over his head a couple of times while your right leg supports his back. On the last stretch, lift him by his arms in order to raise his buttocks slightly off the floor. Now gently but firmly move him forward with your right knee (be careful not to hit his spine). As you do so, turn his body toward the left and lower him, face-down, to the floor. Don't *dump* him, and don't hesitate in the middle of this transition: Be firm and continuous in your movement.

Assume a crawling position and place both hands on his back to begin back techniques (see page 96).

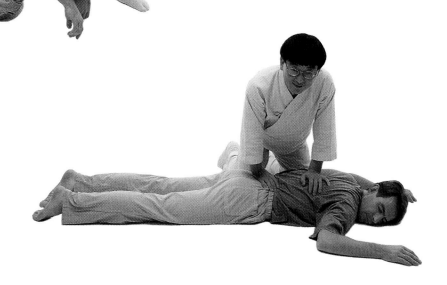

. . . to right-side-up

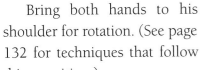

From a standing position behind the receiver, with your right leg supporting his back. Calculate where his head is going to rest and have a pillow in place to support it.

Rotate both his arms and stretch them over his head. During the last stretch, raise his buttocks slightly off the floor, move forward gently with your right knee, turn him toward the left, and lower him onto his left side. Now, grasp his right arm with your left hand, and with your right hand bend his right leg up and move it toward the floor. (Support it with a pillow if the receiver feels a strain in the thigh or back muscles.)

Bring both hands to his shoulder for rotation. (See page 132 for techniques that follow this transition.)

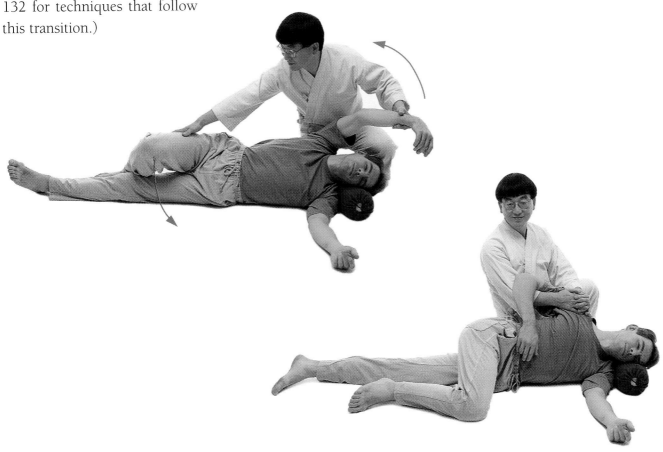

MICRO TRANSITIONS: AN INDEX

Here is a list (including page numbers) of all the micro transitions described in this book.

CHAPTER

SAMPLE

SEQUENCES

LIST OF

BOXED TIPS

Once you have mastered the techniques for changing the receiver's position, you will have all the components necessary for designing your own Ohashiatsu session. You will be able to choose positions and techniques that suit your own capabilities and the receiver's condition, as well as considerations of time and circumstance. The sample sequences that follow not only show combinations of positions, but also selections of techniques to use in each of the positions. An average session takes about 45 minutes to an hour.

When you are designing your own sequences, remember the principles of balance and continuity. Try to work on a yang meridian after a yin meridian, for instance; or follow a center stretch on the neck with a side-to-side stretch. Choose two or three techniques for each part of the body, then go on to an adjacent part. Keep your movements to a minimum but be sure to give yourself enough variety and opportunities for rest. Whenever you, the giver, experience difficulties, fatigue, or discomfort, return to the Kata exercises (Chapter 2) after a session to restore your sense of the basic forms and movements.

Sequence 1.

When the giver is flexible, the receiver is quiet and meditative, and they are already acquainted with each other.

Time: About 40 minutes

FACE-UP
HARA DIAGNOSIS
LEGS AND FEET: Work the Stomach meridian (yang) and two others (one yin and one yang).
ARMS: Work the Heart, Heart Constrictor, and Lung meridians.
NECK: Two gentle techniques; center stretch with four fingers, and stretching in a Figure 8
From face-up to face-down
BACK: Work the Bladder meridian with the palm and thumb.
LEGS: Work the Bladder meridian with the palm and thumb.
From face-down to face-up
FACE AND HEAD: Forehead and neck technique; inner eye technique; temples with the palms; ears with palms and fingers
Return to the hara

Sequence 2.

When the receiver is a pregnant woman who is having her first session and is unknown to the giver.

Time: About 45 minutes

SIT-UP

ARMS: Rotate arms; work three meridians, alternating yin and yang.

BACK: Work the Bladder meridian with the palm and thumb.

Side (right and left)

NECK: Rotate shoulder; work the Gall Bladder meridian in the neck and head.

SHOULDER: Work the Bladder meridian around the shoulder blade.

ARMS: Work the three meridians not worked in the sit-up position.

HIPS: Work the Gall Bladder meridian from the rib cage to the hip.

LEGS: Work the Gall Bladder and Bladder meridians in the upper and lower leg.

Let her rest in side position.

Sequence 3.

When the receiver is overweight and tense, and this is his or her first session; and if the giver is nervous and tired. (Notice that the giver does not face the receiver in this sequence.)

Time: About 40 minutes

FACE-DOWN

BACK: Work the Bladder meridian with the palm only.

LEGS: Work the Bladder meridian with the palm only.

Side (right and left)

NECK: Rotate the shoulder; work the Gall Bladder meridian in the neck and head.

BACK: Work the Bladder meridian around the shoulder blade.

RIBCAGE AND HIP: Work the Gall Bladder meridian from the rib cage to the hip.

LEGS: Work the Gall Bladder and Bladder meridians in the upper and lower leg.

Let him rest in side position.

LIST OF BOXED TIPS

AFTERWORD AND ACKNOWLEDGMENTS

Creating this book has been like writing an autobiography: It keeps reflecting my life. Since I came to America in 1970, I have been practicing and teaching bodywork as a form of healing. For me bodywork is the manifestation of my spirituality. My feelings and beliefs are expressed concretely in my bodywork technique. When I changed my approach and my technique, I changed my inner self. The inner self probably began to change first, but I did not recognize it until I realized it was time to change my method.

When I started practicing bodywork in the United States, I found myself presented with bodies that were much larger than mine, Americans who were skeptical about shiatsu and skeptical about my youth. I felt I had to win over these clients. I pressed hard; I manipulated; I used techniques meant to dazzle and amaze them. But through it all, I didn't feel quite right about myself or what I was doing.

Over a period of two years, I slowly began to change the way I worked. It was difficult to make these changes, but as I did, I began to feel more comfortable with myself. I began to feel less controlled by fear of the receiver and more confident about what I was doing—I stopped worrying about the receiver's reaction—I began to feel *natural*. And the more natural I became, the more the receivers trusted my abilities; as I gained confidence in myself, their confidence in me also increased. I began to enjoy my work much more. My renewed self-confidence allowed me to further modify my approach and technique.

After my book *Do-It-Yourself Shiatsu* was published in 1976, I realized that I was practicing and developing a very different form of bodywork than the one I had written about, and that this difference was growing. So I decided to start keeping records of each new technique in a notebook. After a few years of experimenting, I named my method *Ohashiatsu,* and I started teaching it and asking my students how it worked for them.

In 1990, after I put together a book proposal containing 500 photographs with sample captions, I approached some publishing houses with them. Paul De Angelis, the editor who had first worked with me on another of my books, *Reading the Body,* bought the rights for Kodansha America, and the long process of creating a final manuscript began.

It has not been an easy process for me, partly because of my heavy travel schedule, but also because I found it very difficult to write about techniques that I had previously expressed only verbally and with my body.

In addition, it felt strange to have to decide on definitive techniques and their order, as well as what to emphasize and what not, because every time I teach, I change my curriculum and approach, depending on the experience of the students.

Paul was amazingly astute in the organization of my mass of material. He guided the decision-making process by asking me countless questions and shaping my rambling sentences into coherent paragraphs.

Finally in 1994, with the help of my son, Kazuhiro, I began taking snapshots of all the techniques that I wanted to include in the book. Each technique required two or three shots from different angles, and we took hundreds of pictures. At the same time, I dictated many pages of text, which were expertly transcribed, edited, and organized by Dale Evva Gelfand.

My wife, Bonnie, who used to be a book editor, found the time to draft most of the captions and other text for the main body of this book. We worked day and night and had innumerable discussions and disagreements over the material before Sarah Gearhart appeared, to save my book and my marriage. She completed the captions and other text and, later, guided us through the proofs. Her patience and attention to detail contributed to the quality of the book.

In April and October of 1995, we went into a professional studio to shoot 1,500 photographs with Kan Okano, one of the best photographers in New York City. Okano-san is a true artist, and despite the endless hours of his relentless perfectionism, I was somehow still able to smile for the camera with the assistance of the talented models Mary Hagiwara, Yue Deng, and Igor Titov.

Another welcome addition to the project was Sandy Choron, the original book packager, who brought her discerning eye and warm enthusiasm. In the critical process of converting text and photographs into final layouts, I have been lucky to have the design skills of Matthew Van Fleet, overseen by Kodansha's art and production director, Lucy Hebard, and the keen editorial attention of Kodansha's managing editor, Akiko Takano. Finally, I wish to thank Kodansha's Executive Vice President, Minato Asakawa, for the expert guidance and enthusiasm he maintained throughout the project's development.

My deepest gratitude goes to everyone who contributed to the creation of this book, including the staff at the Ohashi Institute, our dedicated Certified Ohashiatsu® Instructors worldwide, and

our students, who all encouraged me to finish it. Three staff members were particularly helpful with the meridian charts and final proofs: David Coulter, DeeDee Seeley, and my niece, Kumiko Kanayama.

Above all, my wife, Bonnie Harrington Ohashi, is really the mother of all my work, and it is in honor of her nurturing care that I dedicate this book.

Love and health,
OHASHI

Kinderhook, New York, U.S.A.
Spring 1996

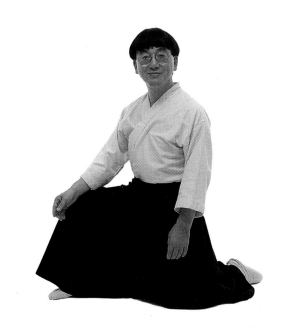

MERIDIAN CHARTS

Using the Meridian Charts

Meridians are pathways of ki energy, and as with other aspects of Eastern thought are classified as yin and yang. The yin meridians travel from bottom to top (earth to heaven) and the yang meridians travel from top to bottom (heaven to earth). In Ohashiatsu we go with the direction of the meridian lines to energize the receiver, and against the direction of the meridian lines to sedate the receiver.

The fourteen meridians and their names were established thousands of years ago by Chinese acupuncturists. Some of the names—for example, the Conception Vessel meridian—may seem strange because they don't correspond to Western anatomical thought. Others whose names refer to body organs in Western terminology are not always related to that organ. These names are based on the ancient Chinese view of human bodily and psychological functions and activity. For example, one function of the body is getting food in order to survive. The meridian that relates to that activity is the Stomach meridian. Another function is providing heat; the Triple Heater meridian relates to that function.

It will help you to know the direction of each meridian and its general location (either the outside or the inside of the leg, for instance), but you do not need to make yourself a "prisoner" of knowing precise locations before you start practicing. Before you study the meridians and their names, learn how to use your body and how to feel the receiver's body—learn from feeling and being.

The meridian charts show the meridians and the major tsubos along them. (The captions tell you if a meridian is yin or yang.) For the beginner, it can sometimes be confusing to read "work up the meridian" or "work down the meridian" when the anatomy or the receiver's position seems to indicate otherwise. For example, when working up the yin meridians in the arms, we are working up the meridian even if the arm is perpendicular to the torso or even pointing downward. Use the charts as guides when you practice the techniques in this book, but don't try to memorize the meridians or worry about their functions until you are thoroughly comfortable with your own movement.

When you are ready for further reading about which meridian lines relate to which health conditions, and to learn more about additional tsubo points, I suggest consulting my books *Do-It-Yourself Shiatsu* and *Reading the Body*.

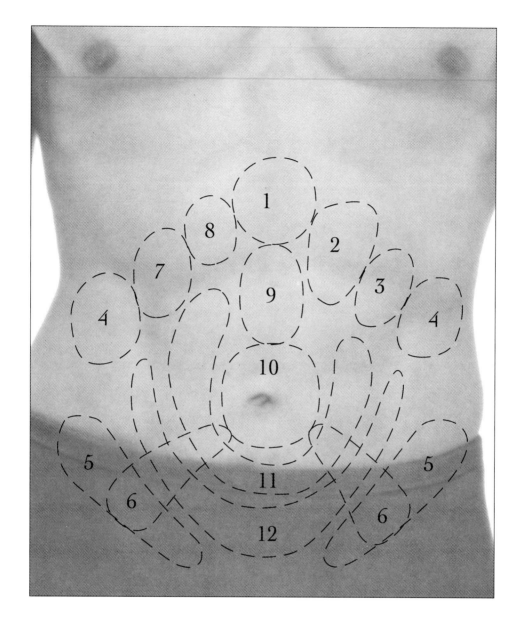

1 Heart	5 Large Intestine	9 Heart Constrictor
2 Stomach	6 Small Intestine	10 Spleen
3 Triple Heater	7 Liver	11 Kidney
4 Lung	8 Gall Bladder	12 Bladder

For the reader's convenience, the hara chart that appears on page 48 of the text is reproduced here. Numbers indicate the recommended order of movement around the hara. Note that some diagnostic areas (Lung, Large Intestine, and Small Intestine meridians) are on both sides of the body. Move in a clockwise direction around the hara (see text page 50 for instruc-

tions), and repeat those diagnostic areas as you come to them. Don't lean into both sides at the same time.

Once you have developed smooth movement when working clockwise around the hara, you can add diagnostic areas 9, 10, 11, and 12 to your routine by working down from the top of the solar plexus, with your left or right hand.

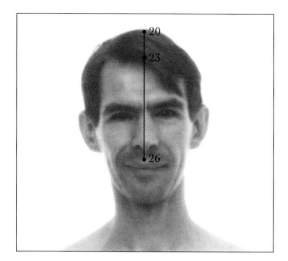

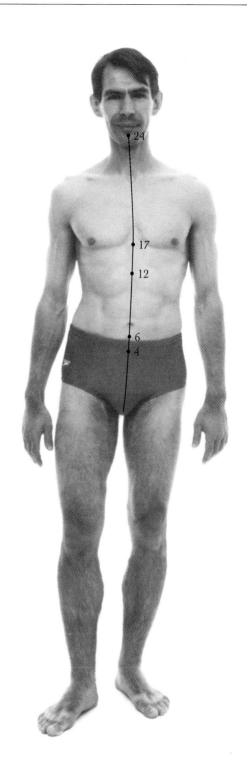

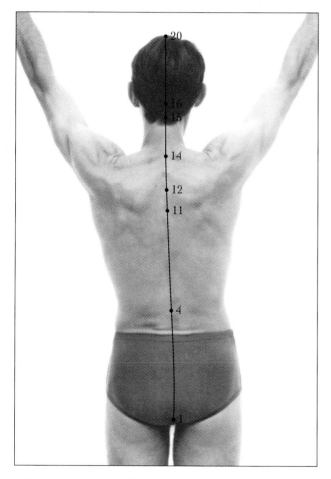

The Governing Vessel meridian is a yang meridian that governs all of the yang meridians. It runs from the middle of the upper lip, up the center of the face, down the back of the head and neck, and down the spine, ending midway between the coccyx and the anus.

The Conception Vessel meridian is a yin meridian that is responsible for all of the yin meridians. It runs from midway between the anus and the scrotum or labia, up the center of the front of the torso and the neck, ending at the middle of the lower lip.

7

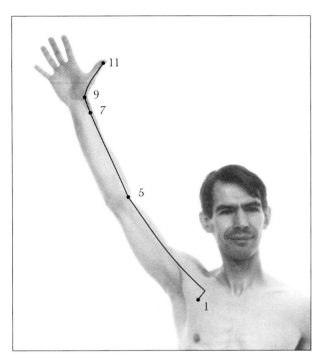

The Lung meridian is a yin meridian associated with the intake of oxygen. It runs from the collarbone along the outside edge of the arm and forearm to the tip of the thumb, just below the nail.

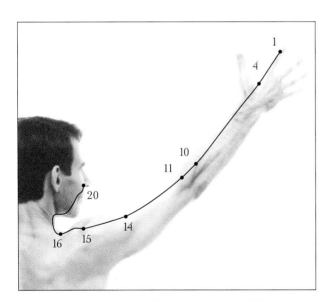

The Large Intestine meridian is a yang meridian associated with the absorption of energy and the elimination of waste. It runs from the tip of the index finger up along the outside edge of the forearm and arm, across the shoulder, and up the throat to the corner of the mouth, ending at the nostril.

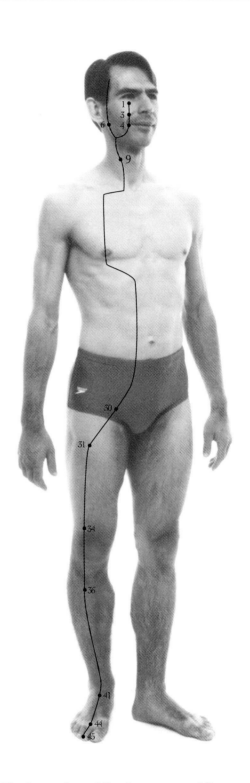

The Stomach meridian is a yang meridian associated with appetite. It runs in two branches down the front and side of the face to the chin, where the branches merge and run down the neck, along the chest, the front of the thigh, and the outside of the shinbone, ending at the tip of the second toe.

2

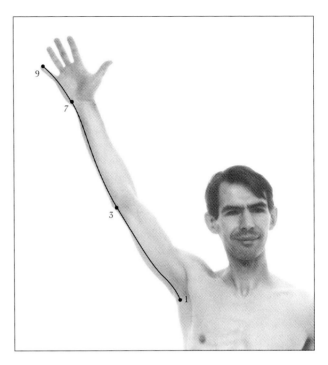

The Heart meridian is a yin meridian associated with circulation and the proper functioning of the heart. It runs from the armpit along the innermost edge of the arm and forearm to the inside of the little finger, just below the nail.

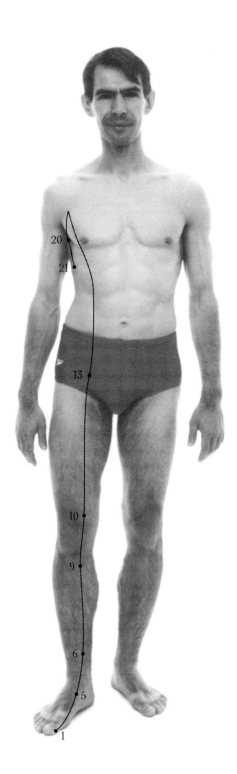

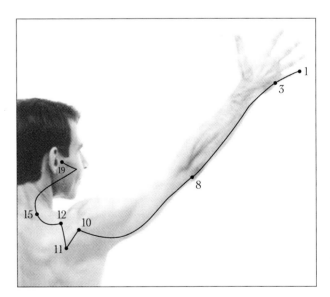

The Spleen meridian is a yin meridian associated with digestion and reproduction. It runs from the big toe up along the inside of the shinbone and the thigh, across the outside edge of the abdomen, up to the armpit, and then down the side of the chest, ending on the side of the sixth rib.

The Small Intestine meridian is a yang meridian associated primarily with the absorption of energy. It runs from the little finger, just below the nail, up the back of the forearm and arm to the shoulder, where it turns down to the shoulder blade, then runs up the neck, ending in front of the earlobe.

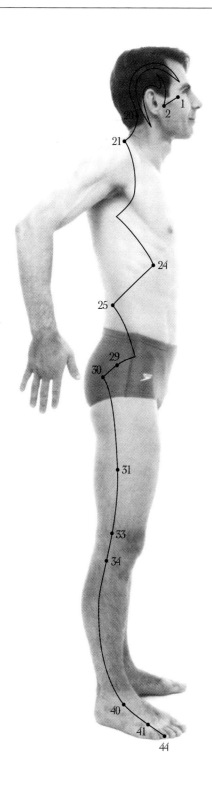

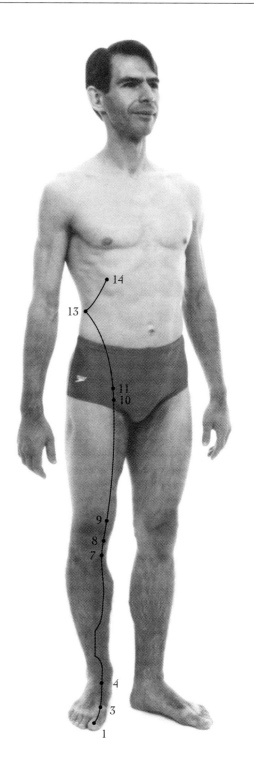

The Gall Bladder meridian is a yang meridian associated with the absorption and distribution of energy. It begins at the temple, runs down around the ear, back up the side of the head to the forehead, down again along the neck and across the shoulder; then it zigzags along the side of the torso and hip, and runs down the outside of the thigh and leg, ending on the fourth toe.

The Liver meridian is a yin meridian associated with the storage and distribution of energy. It runs from the big toe up along the inside of the calf muscle and the thigh, across the abdomen to the bottom of the ribcage and up, ending between the sixth and seventh ribs.

⟨ 6 ⟩

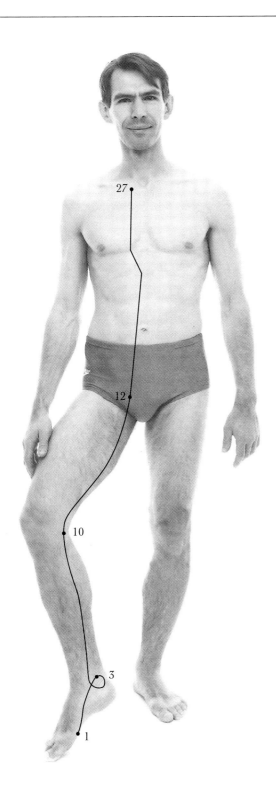

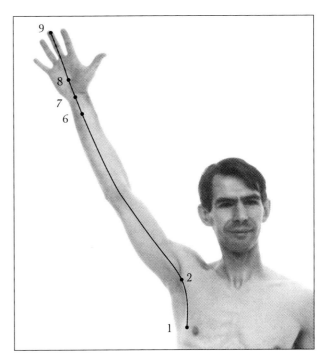

The Heart Constrictor meridian is a yin meridian associated with the pumping of the heart. It runs from the armpit straight down the middle of the arm and forearm (on the inside) to the middle finger.

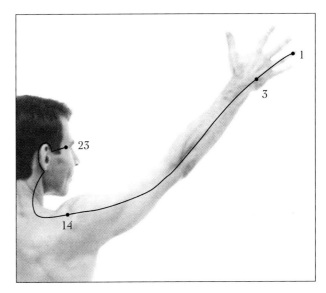

The Kidney meridian is a yin meridian associated with purification and elimination. It runs from the sole of the foot, just below the second and third toes, along the arch, and out and around the ankle; then it runs up the inner edge of the calf muscle, the inside of the thigh, and the center of the torso, ending just below the point where the collarbone meets the sternum.

The Triple Heater meridian is a yang meridian associated with the regulation of temperature and the distribution of energy. It runs from the fourth finger up the back of the forearm and arm, across the shoulder, up the side of the neck, and around the outer edge of the ear, ending at the temple.

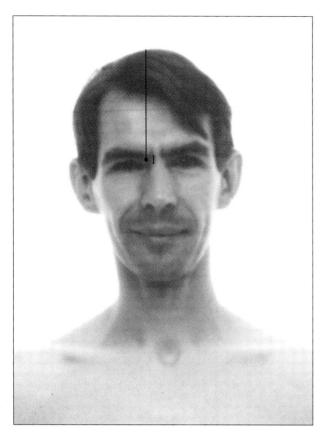

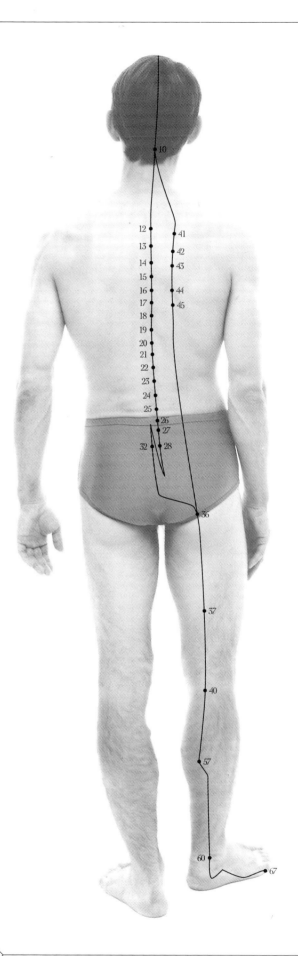

The Bladder meridian is a yang meridian associated with the elimination of waste. It runs from the inner corner of the eye up the forehead and down the back of the head to the base of the neck; there it splits into two branches that run down the back, parallel to the spine, across the buttock, and down the back of the upper leg; at the back of the knee, the two branches merge and continue down the calf, behind the ankle, and along the outside of the foot, ending just below the nail on the outer edge of the little toe.